# THE NATURE OF THE WHOLE

*Holism in Ancient Greek*
*and*
*Indian Medicine*

# INDIAN MEDICAL TRADITION

*Edited by*
DOMINIK WUJASTYK
&
KENNETH G. ZYSK

**Vol. VII**

# THE NATURE OF THE WHOLE

## *Holism in Ancient Greek and Indian Medicine*

VICKI PITMAN

MOTILAL BANARSIDASS PUBLISHERS
PRIVATE LIMITED • DELHI

*First Edition: Delhi, 2006*



ISBN: 81-208-2734-1

MOTILAL BANARSIDASS
41 U.A. Bungalow Road, Jawahar Nagar, Delhi 110 007
8 Mahalaxmi Chamber, 22 Bhulabhai Desai Road, Mumbai 400 026
236, 9th Main III Block, Jayanagar, Bangalore 560 011
203 Royapettah High Road, Mylapore, Chennai 600 004
Sanas Plaza, 1302 Baji Rao Road, Pune 411 002
8 Camac Street, Kolkata 700 017
Ashok Rajpath, Patna 800 004
Chowk, Varanasi 221 001

*Printed in India*
BY JAINENDRA PRAKASH JAIN AT SHRI JAINENDRA PRESS,
A-45 NARAINA, PHASE-I, NEW DELHI 110 028
AND PUBLISHED BY NARENDRA PRAKASH JAIN FOR
MOTILAL BANARSIDASS PUBLISHERS PRIVATE LIMITED,
BUNGALOW ROAD, DELHI 110 007

# CONTENTS

# FOREWORD

It comes as a surprise to learn that the word "holism" was first coined in English in the 20th century by the South African military and political leader, General Jan Christian Smuts (1870-1950). Smuts' 1926 book, *Holism and Evolution* used the term to designate the tendency in nature to produce wholes (i.e. bodies or organisms) from the ordered grouping of unit structures. Since then, many authors have adopted the term which, like *gestalt,* captures the important concept that vital meanings of our world cannot necessarily be understood by an examination of its parts. To put it differently, certain entities have an essence that is indissoluble, that is a result of their wholeness, not of their constituent elements. Or, as the saying goes, "big is different".

Today, the concept of holism is used widely in the field of Complementary and Alternative Medicine (CAM), where it captures the sense that if medical diagnosis and therapy focus merely on the parts of a patient, or on the parts of a disease entity, then a vital part of the medical situation is occluded. There is a wholeness in the situation, in the unity of the patient's whole life and disease state, that is worth attending to. And attention to that wholeness leads—CAM practitioners claim—to a positive transformation in health care and patient management.

Is this concept of holistic medicine a unique development of the 20th century? In the present book, Vicki Pitman dives deep into the Greek tradition of Hippocrates, the father of Western medicine, to discover whether the roots of holism can be found there. If such roots can be found, then perhaps we can say that Modern Establishment Medicine (MEM) has lost something important that it once had, something worth reclaiming in contemporary practice.

But Pitman does not stop at that. The classical medicine of India, Ayurveda, is rapidly undergoing the twin processes of globalisation and modernisation. As such, Pitman recognises it as a medical force on the world stage. And modern, global

Āyurveda also makes the claim to be a holistic medical system. Is that really true? And what exactly does it mean in practice? Pitman returns to the ancient founding documents of Āyurveda, from over two thousand years ago, and searches for the concept and interpretation of holistic medicine in tradition, confronting it comparatively with the evidence from ancient Greece.

Pitman's study is distinguished by several features: originality, scholarly integrity, and accessibility. Perhaps the most important is its historical probity. Pitman grapples with the original texts of Greek and Indian medicine, refusing to simplify, refusing to take anybody else's word for their meaning.

In doing so, Pitman has produced a study which is factually trustworthy, serious, and true to the traditions it explores.

The present series, *Indian Medical Tradition,* is designed to publish exactly this kind of work, which is both scholarly and accessible, both original and topical. Vicki Pitman's reflections and research have much to offer to medical practitioners, medical historians, cultural anthropologists and others. We are delighted and proud to be able to include Vicki Pitman's book in this series.

October 2005 —DOMINIK WUJASTYK

—KENNETH G. ZYSK

# PREFACE

The name Hippocrates is fundamental to Western medicine. He is often quoted but seldom are references given and few today outside the realms of Classical scholarship appreciate the scope or detail of the works. A chance discovery on the shelves of a provincial library of Ludwig Edelstein's Ancient Medicine prompted me to investigate the Hippocratic *Corpus* and its authors. Several aspects of the physician's world Edelstein described seemed so like that of a modern complementary herbal practitioner like myself that I simply wanted to find out more: to see if Hippocratic medicine was the source of our holistic practice and how substantial a record of precept and practice remained that a modern practitioner could draw upon. From the lectures of Dr. Vasant Lad I learned of a sister tradition from India, ancient but still practised, which I felt could help me evaluate and illuminate that of ancient Greece. In the process I found that any notions of boundaries between east and west are actually misleading. Healing arts in many societies draw on universal intimations of holism, human life as part of a greater, spiritual whole.

This book is based on the dissertation for the M. Phil. in Complementary Health Studies at Exeter University (1999). I am very grateful to so many people for their generous aid and guidance. The excellent Centre for Complementary Health Studies, and especially my supervisor Roger Hill gave me the supportive base I needed. John Wilkins and Anne Glazier were my academic tutors for Greek and Ayurvedic medicine; I benefited much and enjoyed much from my discussions with them. Drs. Vasant Lad and Robert Svoboda brought a high standard of Ayurvedic training to western students. Vivian Nutton and Rebecca Fleming generously made time to answer my questions and guide my thoughts about the Hippocratic *Corpus*. My dear friend Dr. Keller Freeman kindly helped with the revision of the dissertation. Sue Williams of Yeovil College Library helped me obtain many needed books without my having to travel, by using the facilities of the marvelous British Library loan service. The Library of the Wellcome Centre for the History of Medicine and its staff were also most valuable and helpful. Lois Reynolds gave generously of her time in the final stages.

Several Ayurvedic physicians kindly allowed me to observe their clinical work and made themselves available for interview: Dr. Deepika Gunawant of London, whom I met through the good offices of Gopi Warrier; Dr. O.P. Arora of Ludhiana and Dr. Gopal Sharma of Jullundhur, Punjab; Dr. J.V.K. Taneja and Dr. Narish Jaiswar of the Ayurvedic and Unani Tibbia College, Karol Bagh, Delhi. Dr. Ram Manohar and his students at ARMARC (Karnataka, India) were good enough to proof the typescript for errors and provide the correct diacritical marks for the Ayurvedic portions of the work. John Wilkins generously did the same for the Greek. I am perhaps most indebted to Dominik Wujastyk. Having read the dissertation, he encouraged me to offer it for publication and facilitated in many ways its preparation. Also, as a person and a scholar he has been an inspiration to me. Finally, I thank Mary Burgess for her support and particularly my husband Tony Pitman, a Classics scholar. His enthusiasm for Greek culture is highly infectious! As I delved into the texts and commentaries, and grappled with Greek words and concepts, he helped in innumerable ways.

—Vicki Pitman

# INTRODUCTION

## ANCIENT GREEK MEDICINE AND CONTEMPORARY HOLISTIC MEDICINE

> Perhaps you too have heard what good doctors say when a patient comes to them with sore eyes. They say, I think, that they cannot attempt to heal his eyes alone, but that they must treat his head too at the same time, if his sight is to recover. They say too that to think that one could ever treat the head by itself without the whole body is quite foolish. On that principle then, they apply their regimens to the entire body and attempt to treat and heal the part in conjunction with the whole. Plato: *Charmides*, 156 b-c.[1]

This fifth century B.C. report of the approach of physicians in ancient Athens towards disease and healing is striking in its similarity to the approach of twentieth century practitioners of complementary, or 'holistic' medicine. Indeed so striking is it that it prompts the questions: Is it possible that the origins for the contemporary holistic approach are to be found in 'that principle' on which these ancient Greek physicians based their work? What else is there in their work which is still either germane to, or reflected in, the practice of present day holistic medicine?

Answers to such questions are important for several reasons. Many contemporary holistic practitioners are attracted to study the traditional and ancient medical systems of, for example China, India, Tibet, or Native Americans precisely because they offer an integrated approach to health care (both cure and prevention) grounded in a comprehensive understanding of living beings. Such systems are perceived from the outset to be 'holistic' and it is this quality that their Western practitioners perhaps feel is

1. Saunders *et al.* (1987) 180.

lacking within a Western context. It is the aim of this thesis to establish whether or not there is a tradition for holism native to Europe and comparable to these systems in its comprehensiveness.

Of course many practitioners and even many laypersons may be vaguely aware that they are working within a tradition traceable back to ancient times. For example, they may quote snippets of Hippocrates, or perhaps more rarely Galen, but the totality of the tradition such figures represent is not as immediate or well-known to them as the tradition of ancient Ayurvedic writers is for contemporary *vaidyas* (physicians).[2] Among practitioners, there seems a far larger proportion of concepts congenial to holistic medicine which are borrowed or incorporated from non-European medical traditions.[3] Teaching introductory classes of herbal medicine to the general public, this author has found that the concept of yin and yang, of five phases, is much more widely known than that of the elements, temperaments and humours of the Greco–Roman, pre-Enlightenment world. Āyurveda is similarly enjoying at present a wide exposure in the popular media.

The appeal of these systems seems to lie in the fact that they are at one time both ancient and modern. Their origin is in the ancient world and they have continued to exist, one way or another, throughout the centuries, to grow and develop, to have withstood the onslaught of colonialism and to continue to be practised efficaciously down to the present day. Though

---

2. The reasons for this distance are many. Partly it may be due to such factors as lack of general education in ancient history or ancient languages, partly to the fact of growing up in a culture wedded to the scientific method, which implies a rejection of truths and solutions from a pre-scientific time and in which the physical body has for a long period of time been viewed as dissociated from human consciousness.
3. R. Coward (1989) 36, has pointed out that "'the East' has a privileged position in these philosophies, [and] carries this automatic advantage...they carry the implication of ancient truths, based on a 'true' understanding of nature, and sometimes linked with religions. Thus any oriental therapy carries this automatic advantage. Based on systems long used in China, India and the Far East, they carry the implication of ancient and traditional wisdoms which have a much closer relation to the body and natural instincts than anything produced in the West."

certainly not unchanged throughout their history, the integrity of their grounding in tradition remains intact.

By contrast, the concepts and practices of what might be termed traditional European medicine are less well known and connected to the day-to-day practice of contemporary holistic medicine practitioners. We are less aware of being part of a tradition going back some two thousand years than is an Indian Ayurvedic *vaidya*.

## PURPOSE AND METHODOLOGY

The questions which are prompted therefore are: Is this lack of connection to a Western tradition of holistic medicine due to the absence in the ancient science of medicine of anything which is valid today for today's practitioners? Or perhaps is it due to the absence of a 'western' holistic model of sufficient substance to understand health and treat disease? In attempting to answer these questions, this book examines the Hippocratic *Corpus* from the point of view of contemporary holistic criteria to ascertain if there is a corresponding model for understanding and treating health and disease holistically, of comparable substance to that of holistic models from other traditions. The Hippocratic *Corpus* is chosen because it is the most extensive written record of the ancient European ideas about medicine and health, forming the major starting point of Galen's system, which itself became the dominant model for health and care until the scientific revolution.

Extensive quotations from the *Corpus* are given in order that the writers may speak for themselves as often as possible. Even with this, the effort is not without its dangers. As Wesley Smith has remarked in his introduction to his translations of the *Epidemics* (Books 2, 4-7) each subsequent commentator or scholar of the *Corpus* beginning with Galen himself has tended to read into the works the prevailing themes and concerns of himself and his times.[4]

In order to test whether the practices of these ancient physicians and the rationale for those practices still hold any

4. Smith (1994) 9. See also (1979) 14, ff.

validity for modern practitioners, the model of Ayurvedic medicine has been chosen for comparison. Āyurveda will serve as a form of template against which to measure key aspects of the ideas and practices found in the Hippocratic writings. Āyurveda is selected because it originates in the same period of history as the Hippocratic *Corpus*, and is based on a comparable model of bodily 'humours' called *doṣas*. As the main system of traditional medicine in India, regulated by the Indian government and incorporated into its health care system, it is being used by tens of thousands of people as their primary health care system. Traditional medicine systems such as Āyurveda have been recognised as very important parts of health care and the World Health Organisation supports research and training in safe and effective use of traditional medicines such as those of Āyurveda.[5] It thus provides a contemporary model of continuity in a holistic health care system. If sufficient correspondences in ideas and methods exist in the origins of the traditions, this would demonstrate that the rationale and methods of treatment employed by the ancient Greek physicians are not just important or interesting relics of the past but are capable of application for effective healing in the present. Finally, by discussing similar concepts common to the two systems and pointing out their differences as well as similarities, I hope to have minimized the tendency to inject contemporary ideas into the *Corpus*.

## Primary Sources

Ancient Greek: The principle text used for this study is the translation of W.H.S. Jones for the Loeb Classical Library, recently enlarged by additional translations by Paul Potter and Wesley Smith.[6] The works of the *Corpus* will be referred to by their titles as translated by Jones, Potter and Smith, e.g. *Nutriment*. Chapters and passages within the treatises cited will similarly follow the identifications of these translators, e.g.

5. WHO Traditional Medicine Programme, 1977 and Progress Report on Traditional Medicine and Modern Health Care, 1991.
6. Only Volume III covering fractures, wounds in the heads, and joints, has not been studied in detail as containing less directly relevant material.

the Roman enumeration of Jones or the Arabic of Potter and Smith.

Some use is also made of *Anonymus Londinensis*, translated by W.H.S. Jones, and of translations of *The Seed* and *The Nature of the Child* by I. Lonie in *Hippocratic Writings*, edited by G.E.R. Lloyd.

Ancient Indian: The text of Āyurveda is that of *Caraka Saṃhitā*, compiled in the first century A.D. *Caraka* has been chosen because, although later than the Hippocratic writings, many of its concepts and methods are now believed to derive from the more ancient medical practices, of the sixth and fifth centuries B.C. Therefore the two texts seem suitable for the purposes of comparison.

The translation used is that of R.K. Sharma and *Vaidya* (Doctor) Bhagwan Dash and includes the most influential historical commentary on the text by the eleventh century writer Cakrapāṇidatta.

## Secondary Sources

The Hippocratic *Corpus* was at one time studied and read by many bio-medical physicians who, while no longer concerned to practise its methods, drew inspiration from it in other ways. It has also been subject to extensive research by scholars in the Classics. Their studies and commentaries are a chief resource for this present research. However, it is recognised that their viewpoint is necessarily shaped by the prevailing world view of their times and their conclusions are similarly shaped. For example, for a period many scholars were concerned to find in the *Corpus* the seeds of the post-Enlightenment scientific method and any feature which pointed to this was discussed prominently, while other aspects, such as the concepts underpinning treatment and the practical healing methods were given limited consideration or discussed for historical purposes only.[7] More recently, interest in the *Corpus* has revived and studies have

---

7. Examples of this attitude are found in the introductions to the treatises in the Loeb edition by its translator, W.H.S. Jones. For a survey of the various ways in which the treatises have been interpreted and used by later writers, see Smith (1979) 14-41.

begun to concentrate more on questions of "what they, the ancients themselves, thought they were doing. That is the key question...."[8] This approach is very welcome to the present study.

However, few if any of these scholars are practitioners treating patients and their maladies. According to Smith, the last scholar for whom the *Corpus* was relevant to current medical practice was M.P.E. Littré, who was himself a physician. Reading Hippocrates in his own image and that of the medicine of his time, Littré was the "last commentator for whom Hippocrates was alive and meaningful in day to day medical practice."[9] For practitioners of holistic medicine, there is some disadvantage in relying on scholars for translation, interpretations and historical background. This is another reason why the use of a comparison with a similar system which is still practised, such as Āyurveda, can help to extend and balance the practitioner's understanding of the *Corpus*.

The ancient Sanskrit medical texts such as *Caraka* have not received to the same extent the critical scholarship given to the Greek. Critical appraisal began with Julius Jolly's *Indian Medicine* (1901), a historical and orderly discussion of the texts and relevant literature on Āyurveda. Jean Filliozat's *The Classical Doctrine of Indian Medicine* was the next major contribution and since the 1970s more work has begun to appear, much of it published in journals such as *The Journal of the European Ayurvedic Society*, or from symposia such as the International Workshop on the Study of Indian Medicine (1985).[10] Dominik Wujastyk's forthcoming *Sanskrit Medical Writings* will be a welcome addition to the field. To such sources is added information on historical background from scholarship on the history of Indian philosophies and Indian cultural history. There have been many books published in the last decade on Āyurveda, both by Indian and Western Ayurvedic

8. Lloyd (1994) 27.
9. Smith (1979) 31. See also Smith (1994) vol. VII 9. "Thus we read ourselves into these works."
10. Papers published as *Studies on Indian Medical History* (1987) Muelenbeld and Wujastyk.

physicians or interested lay persons. However, there is difficulty in using them for the present study because they draw on the whole of Ayurvedic tradition, rather than *Caraka Saṃhitā* only, and are less concerned with the history of ideas. However, in relying only on scholars, again from the practitioner's point of view, some relevance to practice is lost. Thus as an exception, *Āyurveda: Life, Health and Longevity* by Robert Svoboda has been consulted, and some use has been made of lecture material by Dr. Vasant Lad. In addition, in order to corroborate the continued existence of ancient medical practices in contemporary settings, observations and interviews were conducted at an Ayurvedic clinic in London and at a government Ayurvedic training college and clinic in New Delhi.

Before setting out to examine our sources for holistic elements, it is important to discuss what the terms 'holistic' or 'holism' mean.

## HOLISM AND HOLISTIC MEDICINE

For the purposes of this paper 'holistic' medicine is that approach to understanding and treating health and disease which endeavours to be inclusive of the complex of factors and relationships which make up the human being. As such it stands in contrast to that of the prevailing orthodoxy of 'bio-medicine', which is more exclusively physically based and organised around separation, reduction and specialisation.[11]

11. It is recognised that due to the changes from within conventional medicine in recent years, the lines of demarcation between the two approaches are beginning to blur. For example, many of the ideas of holistic medicine are now embraced by orthodox medicine, and that, moreover, the traditional debate in medicine between the 'art' and 'science' of medicine reflects the fact that there have always been individual physicians who have understood and treated more 'holistically', with due attention to the mental and spiritual needs of their patients. The Peckham Experiment in the 1930s and 1940s is another example of such an approach. On the other side, herbalists and massage therapists, for example, are keen to use scientific understanding to validate their practices. Nevertheless the dominant health care system favours a high degree of specialisation, with less attention to the individuality of disease processes. Each specialist still is responsible only for that part of the patient which he is trained to treat, thus maintaining a reductionist approach. Moreover, holism is the

Holistic has also been used synonymously with 'natural' medicine, 'alternative' medicine, and 'complementary' medicine.[12] Implicit in each of these epithets is an attempt to differentiate it from bio-medicine.

'Natural' indicates that such methods used are based on naturally-occurring substances or human touch, as opposed to machine technology. These include, for example, both herbs and dietary therapies, and non-invasive manual techniques such as massage or manipulation, ones requiring nothing other than human to human touch and rudimentary mechanical or chemical technology. The term is problematic in that many naturally-occurring plant substances are poisonous. Just because something is natural, it is not automatically safe. Further, it tends to create a false dichotomy between man and nature. However, what is relevant in the use of 'natural' is the attempt to indicate that any therapy tries to work with and within the naturally-occurring forces, cycles, and processes of the natural world and the human body, and to which the body's functions are adapted.

'Alternative' is a term used to indicate that such approaches are offered or chosen as an alternative to the dominant medical model. 'Complementary' is a term often used by those who view the relationship with the dominant model less antagonistically and more inclusively, or who feel that the approach can be included as an addition to complement, or 'complete' the whole of health care delivered. 'Integrated health care' is a term that is currently being suggested as describing an inclusive system in which both the less orthodox and orthodox medical disciplines are made available to the patient.[13]

Holistic medicine has most commonly and perhaps most briefly been defined as that approach which includes 'body,

---

premise and starting point of holistic medicine, whereas this is not the case with the dominant medical model. For other discussions of the differences between bio-medicine and holistic medicine see: Featherstone and Forsyth *Medical Marriage* (1997) and Pietroni *The Greening of Medicine* (1990).

12. Pietroni maintains that bio-medicine can be "holistic", 25-26.
13. See *Integrated Health Care* (1997).

mind and spirit'. With some exceptions, whereas orthodox medicine views health and disease primarily within purely physical parameters, is highly reductive and specialised, and bases treatment almost exclusively on drug, surgical or other technological interventions, holistic medicine starts from a different premise. It holds that although disease has physical manifestation, its origins are not exclusively physical or due exclusively to exogenous pathogens, or to genetics. Therefore an exclusively physical approach does not address the root causes of the disease, sometimes a complex of factors, nor bring about the most complete resolution. Holistic medicine attempts to understand the patient within a wider 'whole' and its therapeutic methods attempt to treat individual aspects of this whole in concert with this greater whole.

The term holistic in fact comes from the Greek word *holos* meaning whole. There is a close linguistic association between wholeness and wellness. The origin of our words 'health' and 'heal' lies in the Germanic/old English *hael*, or whole.[14] Being whole and healthy or healed can in fact be seen as that which occurs when the parts are well integrated and well co-ordinated within the whole, all co-operating towards its well-being. In the Hippocratic treatises there is no discussion or definition of the term, since the physicians were not self-consciously holistic, as opposed to reductionist. But even for them the wholeness seems to hold particular interest. The relationship between the parts and the whole is often mentioned.

There are several characteristic attributes or premises of holistic medicine as it is understood today by such diverse disciplines as herbal medicine, osteopathy, naturopathy, aromatherapy and reflexology, which give definition to this complementary approach.[15]

---

14. *Collins English Dictionary* (1995) 699, 717.
15. Pietroni, a founder of the British Holistic Medicine Association, has described the changes in scientific and medical thinking which have influenced him and other medical doctors and nurses. In *The Greening of Medicine* (1990), 16-27, he traces the history of the holistic concept from J. C. Smutts (*Holism and Evolution*) whom he credits with its first use in modern times, through contemporary scientists such as Lovelock (the 'Gaia Hypothesis') and Weiss and Von Bertanfly (General Systems Theory).

## Vital Force

The concept of a vital force is the recognition that there is a force or energy within the natural world, and thus within the human body, responsible for life. Such a force is not necessarily material, although it is implicit in material forms. It is sometimes referred to as subtle. While perhaps not as yet measurable by physical means, nevertheless it is acknowledged to exist and to be imbedded in and to influence the physical level of reality and vice versa.[16] It is sometimes called the universal life-force. It is considered to be found in all forms in this universe, animate and inanimate, though at varying degrees of activity. It is considered to be intelligent and intelligible as reflected in the orderliness of the world; even chaos theory has its own internal logic. Those of a religious disposition may choose to attribute the source of this vital force to God or Christ, but others may call it simply Nature or the Creative Power.[17]

This vital force or energy is optimal and beneficial when it flows freely and in a balanced way through the body and is not blocked or congested in any particular part or area. To the extent to which it becomes blocked, congested or otherwise disrupted, its life and health enhancing influence is diminished and this is the basic source of disease. Such

16. For example, for thousands of years electricity was not known to exist, even denied, until sufficient understanding and instrumentation was developed to measure and harness it.

17. Examples of this premise held by practitioners of holistic medicine can be found in the works of, for example, John Lust, Dr. John Christopher, Michael Tierra, and Dr. H.C. Vogel. Earlier examples include Father Kniepp, Samual Hahnemann. Simon Mills feels that 'vitalism' is too much associated with the vitalism vs. mechanistic paradigm of the nineteenth century and that vitalism's implication of an extrinsic causal force which cannot be defined by any criterion is unhelpful. He finds another term more meaningful for today's practitioner: the 'organicism' of Leibniz and Whitehead—"all entities at all levels behave in accordance with their position in the greater pattern of which they are parts'—which seems in fact similar to Smutts" holism. See Mills, *Out of the Earth* (1991), 119-121. The problem is that such positions fail to explain the origin of the 'organicism' in the first place. Mills does make use of Chinese medicine which itself proposes a fundamental principle or *tao* as the origin of the world.

blockage or congestion, it is recognised, may be caused not only by physical factors but as well, or even initially, by thoughts, mental attitudes and emotions. In other words, the human organism is a unity of body, mind and spirit, each interacting and influencing the others profoundly.

## The Wisdom of the Body

The human organism is intelligent and has inherent self-healing abilities. Even the symptoms of disease represent the body's attempt to make the best of an imbalanced situation and to resolve a 'dis-ease'. It follows that methods of treatment, even while preventing damaging progress of an illness, will aim to support and encourage what the body is naturally trying to do: eliminate imbalance. This is the basis of lasting health.

## The Mind-Spirit-Body Connection

Given an underlying vital force behind and within all phenomena, the holistic approach recognises *from the outset* the interconnection between the mind and the body. Here mind is understood to include mental and emotional processes and experiences. The mind is understood as a more subtle, more intelligent manifestation of the same vital force. By extension, the spirit is an even more subtle aspect. Thus there is really no separation between mind and body. That the mind and/or spirit influences the physical body either towards or away from disease, and vice versa, is accepted as fundamental. In treatment the mental–emotional aspect is addressed as well as the physical.[18]

Because the same vital force is within all of our natural world, we are intimately connected to and influenced by all aspects of our environment. This environment includes our social, emotional and physical environment.

---

18. There has developed more recently much medical and scientific interest in the mind–body connection, as the new discipline of *psycho-neuro immunology* attests.

## Health and Disease

Health is understood as a balance of the flow of the vital force and of the body's functions which ensures optimal energy for living and creativity. In a sense, all the varieties of disease that we find are really a variation on one disease, the disharmony of the vital force, its imbalance. This imbalance manifests itself in particular places and with particular symptoms according to the nature of the individual body's congestions or disruptions. Symptoms are a sign of imbalance and not necessarily the disease itself. At the same time the symptoms also represent the body's attempts to right that imbalance, or to contain its damage. It is for this reason that, if possible, symptoms are not to be suppressed, for then the signal of imbalance, which the symptoms represent is merely being ignored, producing more complex imbalance.

## Treatment to Support and Rebalance the Body

Holistic medicine puts as much emphasis on prevention as it does on cure, affirming that a healthy body is less susceptible to disease and can recover from disease more quickly. It is not satisfied with the disappearance of symptoms, but wishes to return the organism and the patient to a solid foundation of health.

A corollary of this is that the methods of healing used are based on the idea that encouraging the positive functioning of all the body's parts is the key to real healing. It is for this reason that, treatment is not limited to suppressing or blocking symptoms; the holistic practitioner works to eliminate them by eliminating their origins in imbalance within the whole system. The practitioner examines the client to discover if the origin is in the mental, emotional or physical sphere, or a combination of these, (e.g. too much uric acid in the system can cause gout. A holistic approach would be to endeavour to calm any inflammation but also to eliminate the excess uric acid from the body, to cleanse or improve the function of the kidneys and to address any aspects of the patient's diet and mental attitudes which are felt to be contributing to the build up of uric acid.)

In a sense the process of healing is the reversal of the progress of the disease. As the organism returns to a more healthy balance, it may undergo a series of crises or turning points in which the body is activated and displays symptoms. But these symptoms are seen in a positive light, as evidence that it is engaged in rebalancing itself. Such healing symptoms may include fevers, which increase the temperature and provoke sweating, skin rashes, increased bowel function, increased urination, or sweating.

## Treat the Individual, not the Disease

Each individual is recognised as a unique manifestation of the universal vital force, with his or her own pattern of strengths and weaknesses, and subject to unique sets of influences from the environment. Diagnosis attempts to understand the particular circumstances of and influences on the patient, and treatment is guided toward these individual characteristics. In practical terms this means, for example, not necessarily giving the same treatment or remedy for a headache to any two people, since the fundamental, underlying cause may be different in each. The aim is to understand why that particular person has the particular type of headache she does, and to treat that person accordingly.

A corollary of this position is that ultimately it is the individual who bears a major share of responsibility for his or her own health. This responsibility is met by an effort to live in reasonable harmony, rather than in conflict with one's relations, environment and inherent balance or pattern of energy. This understanding encourages the patient and the physician to give considerable attention to factors which may have predisposed the organism towards disease, factors which can come from 'outside' the organism (diet, lifestyle, environment, weather) as well as from 'inside' (emotions, thoughts, exercise).

The above characteristics of holistic medicine have been found expressed in numerous forums and media. Most recently *Medical Marriage*, by Featherstone and Forsyth, has sought to outline the distinctions in approach between the bio-medical and holistic models, without discussing the question of origins. The authors distinguish holistic medicine by the following criteria:

> Responding to the person as a whole (body, mind and spirit) within the context of their environment (family, culture, and ecology)...
> A willingness to use a wide range of interventions, from drugs and surgery to meditation and diet...
> An emphasis on a more participatory relationship between doctor and patient...
> An awareness of the impact of the 'health' of the practitioner on the patient (physician heal thyself.)[19]

This paper will attempt to examine the Hippocratic *Corpus* for evidence that such ideas were present in the minds of its authors and shaped their practice. In this we will be looking to a certain extent with somewhat biased eyes in the sense that we will be examining the text from the holistic point of view, the point of view of a practitioner for whom it yet may be 'alive and meaningful' in day-to-day practice, and to be alert to any evidence of holism, not only in theory but in practice. As with recent scholarship in Classics which is re-examining its source to discover the contributions and the situations of women in the ancient world, the attempt here is to re-examine the medical sources for the origins of a holistic medical tradition in Western culture and evaluate them in the light of contemporary holistic understanding.

The book starts with a chapter placing the texts of Caraka and the Hippocratic *Corpus* within their respective historical and philosophical contexts. The nature of the texts themselves is also described. Chapter Two is a brief general survey of concepts in *Caraka* and the *Corpus* which are in harmony with the holistic approach. Each of the next two chapters examines in more depth and detail one concept important to both the medical systems and which exemplifies the holistic approach of the physicians: food and digestion, and the humoral model. A final chapter offers a discussion of the implications of the results of the research for a contemporary holistic pracititioner and the insights gained from comparing the two systems.

19. Featherstone and Forsyth. (1997) 24-27.

CHAPTER 1

# HISTORICAL BACKGROUND TO ANCIENT MEDICINE AND PHILOSOPHY

The Hippocratic *Corpus* is a group of treatises written by physicians of the fifth and fourth centuries B.C. They give us the first extensive written record of the origins of the medical art in Europe. When assessing these writings as to whether they reveal what a contemporary practitioner would recognise as a holistic view of health and disease, it is first important to be aware of the context in which they were written.

Hippocrates is recognised as the father of medicine in European tradition. Until the scientific revolution this referred to the prevailing model of Galenic medicine. He was renowned in his own lifetime, and even in ancient times many legends grew up around his name. The treatises in the *Corpus* were attributed to him. After the development of the scientific method and the dramatic discoveries of modern science, Hippocrates' paternity was transferred to Western scientific medicine in general, and the treatises were gradually read less by practising physicians than by Classics scholars or historians of science. There has been a tendency to look for and find in them the foundations of our modern medicine. Now that holistic medicine has begun to be recognised as a truly complementary body of knowledge with its own methodology it seems time to re-evaluate ancient Western medicine from a fresh point of view. Holistic practitioners in the West may have grounds to claim Hippocrates as the 'father of holistic medicine'.

There was an historical Hippocrates who taught and practised on the island of Cos in around 450 B.C. His fame is attested to by contemporaries such as Plato. However, it has proved impossible to know for certain which treatises, if any, are written by this Hippocrates himself, though W.H.S. Jones, the works' primary English translator, believes certain documents must be by the same author, probably Hippocrates. This question has vexed scholars to our own day. Jones believes the *Corpus* represents the remains of a library, probably that of a medical 'school' at Cos. Anything more is mere conjecture.[1]

The *Corpus* itself comprises about sixty treatises by many different authors. Some are believed to have been written by Hippocrates or his pupil and son-in-law, Polybus. Many others are by various authors, dating between *c.*430 and *c.*330 B.C. with a few slightly later works, dating to *c.*260 B.C. They are all written in Ionian dialect, the same as that used by the Presocratic philosophers. Some are considered to be polemical and rhetorical works defending a particular theory of medicine or persuading an audience of the value of medicine as worthy art and craft. Others are simply case notes recording the progress of diseases in individuals. Some are thought to be lectures or information for the training of student physicians. They were produced in an era when speech was still the pre-eminent means of communication and the nature of writing itself was undergoing dramatic change as it developed from being primarily expressed in poetic to prose forms. There is no complete agreement among the various authors on either the causes or treatments of disease, though there are general points of agreement (or at least underlying assumptions) about disease and wellness displayed in the most authoritative of the treatises.[2]

Jones characterises them as having: (1) a religious element generally discarded; (2) a philosophic element still strong; and (3) a rational element relying on accurate observation and accumulated experience, which concluded that disease and health depended on environment and the constitution of the person.[3]

---

1. Jones (1972) vol. I xxix.
2. Ibid., xx, xxi.
3. Ibid., xiv.

## PHILOSOPHICAL BACKGROUND TO IDEAS AND THEMES FOUND IN THE TREATISES

As has been noted by many scholars, and emphasised most recently by James Longrigg in his book, *Greek Rational Medicine*, Hippocratic writings were inextricably linked to broader philosophical currents of the time. Indeed Longrigg states that Hippocratic medicine 'without the background of Ionian rationalism is inconceivable'. He is refering to the sixth century B.C., during which time, what G.E.R. Lloyd calls a 'revolution of wisdom' had occurred.[4] Lloyd is here applying to the ancient world Thomas Kuhn's idea of sequences of scientific revolutions which replace one paradigm or gestalt with another in the history of modern science. In the previous archaic period, explanations for the various phenomena of life, including disease and death, were sought in the supernatural—gods, goddesses, demons and superheroes. With the Ionian pre-Socratic philosophers and with Pythagoras, explanations began to be sought and found with reference to the world of nature rather than the separate world of gods and goddesses, heroes and demons. This world was open to understanding by means of the observation of physical phenomena and the application of rational analysis.[5]

4. Longrigg (1993) 99. Longrigg's view is that this link was ultimately detrimental to the development of science and medical science overall, albeit with some benefits. Lloyd (1978, 41-44) agrees. He cites such benefits as the innovation of rational observation, the laying of the foundations of knowledge, awareness of methodological issues. Yet in another work Lloyd (1987, 116-119) also characterises other aspects as 'highly schematic', 'drastically over-simplified pathological, therapeutic and physiological doctrines' which ignore the 'manifest controversiality of the subject' and that overstate their case with 'incontestible assertions'. Jones (1972 vol. I, xxiii) felt the main task of Greek medicine was to free science from superstition and from 'philosophical hypotheses'.
5. The word 'rational' is somewhat problematic in our current situation for two reasons. Firstly in recent years, some writers in holistic medicine have attributed the approach of allopathic medicine to disease as stemming from the rationalism of Descartes and the scientific revolution of the 17th century. The implication seems to be, or can be drawn mistakenly, that rational thought is not involved in traditional or natural medicine, that it was totally experiential, intuitive and empirical. Secondly, until very recently, Western scholars writing on traditional medicine whether Greek, Indian or Chinese, have tended to term anything within it that was not in some way a prototype or precursor of our modern scientific medicine or method as unworthy of value; it was dismissed as ineffective, or superstitious, even those aspects which reflect a rational approach. As examples, see Lloyd (1987) 116, 130; (1979), 21-22, 149, 24, 251-252.

Thus the flowering of Greek thought of the sixth, fifth and fourth centuries B.C. the time of the Hippocratic writers, occurred as a major change in *weltangschauung*, at least among a significant portion of the literate, educated citizens. A new paradigm was gradually created and for many subsequent centuries offered a satisfactory explanation for the widest variety of phenomena, Kuhn's definition for a successful paradigm.[6] Although there were disagreements among the thinkers as to details, the general outline of the paradigm, the discovery of 'nature', can be described as follows.

Nature is essentially orderly and regular. Nature itself is divine. Natural phenomenon can be explained by what we observe occurring in this orderly world. This order unfolds according to a certain *arche* or first principle(s), through an intelligent vital force, or life-giving energy. The changes we experience are due to the interaction of the basic elements, having certain qualities or powers, *dunameis*. These basic elements are air, fire, water, earth. Sometimes a fifth element, ether/*aither*, is designated and refers to the more rarefied atmosphere or air of the heavens, or that sphere of the cosmos where heavenly bodies, the sun, moon, stars, and planets, orbit. Their harmonious mingling of the elements in proper proportions, or their disharmony, constitutes the forms and changes to those forms which we experience. These elements were seen to exist and operate both in the external environment and within the human body. In the body they exist as our basic humours, or fluids—bile, phlegm, blood and black bile (a slightly later designation in the *Corpus*). Thus there is an important and inherent macrocosm-microcosm relationship between man and his environment. Such new ideas were born out of the flowering of thought in the sixth and fifth centuries B.C. originating in Miletus on the eastern coast of modern Turkey.

## The Milesian Philosophers of the Sixth Century B.C.

Miletus was one of the three major cities of the colony established by Ionians, an early tribe of Greeks inhabiting the

---

6. Kuhn (1962) 64.

mainland, who, fleeing the Dorian invasions, settled Asia minor from the mainland from about 800 B.C. Because of their literacy, industry and the agricultural fertility of the area, these Greeks, living in city states, prospered and created a highly developed civilisation lasting up to the fifth century. Miletus, positioned near the centre of east-west trade routes benefited from contacts with both Egypt and Persia. Its citizens were politically free and able to travel widely. Milesian culture reached its height in the sixth century with the achievements of its thinkers, artists and poets. From our point of view they are considered among the first rationalists. These thinkers coined the term 'philosophy' for their activities.

What was the nature of this philosophy? We must try to remember that the word did not have quite the same meaning for these ancients as it does for us today. Its long use means it has taken on several associated meanings. Strictly speaking, it comes from two Greek words 'philo', to love, and 'sophia', wisdom, thus in essence its meaning is love of wisdom. Wisdom itself can be defined as the understanding of what is right, true and lasting. Love of wisdom can be said to be a dedication to obtain such understanding and the practical discipline to live according to it. In this original sense, it does not have today's connotations of an academic activity somewhat remote from the problems of daily life, concerned only with what to the lay person would seem obscure or irrelevant ideas. It was originally seen as a striving after what is true and lasting which was also practical and down-to-earth.

Rather than being separated from their society by an academic ivory tower, these earliest Ionian philosophers were known to be practical men of affairs, involved in the political and economic life of their great city. They were applying their minds to solving problems that confronted everyone: What causes an earthquake, a thunderstorm? Was it Zeus hurling a thunderbolt or was there another possible explanation? And instead of attributing these phenomena to the work of gods, they realised they could be explained by natural causes, observable and understandable by human thought. Thales, for example, measured the height of the pyramids, predicted eclipses, and offered an explanation of earthquakes which made no mention of Zeus. He and the other Milesian philosophers were "canonised for their practical wisdom and statesmanship rather than for philosophy in our sense of the word"[7] by the next and subsequent generations of Greeks. Thus, for those living at that time it would seem that explanations of the universe and man's place in it were not separated from daily problems of life.

For us looking back over two thousand years these philosophers are seen to mark a major turning point in development of Western thought and civilisation. Instead of finding an explanation of the universe and physical phenomenon, i.e. of 'life', through reference to non-human forces such as anthropomorphized deities and supernatural demons, they sought to understand and explain phenomena through a study of natural forces, for the most part without reference to gods. Hence the term they used for themselves and their activity was *phusikon*, the study of 'phusis' or nature. As a corollary, human life potentially could now be viewed as free from magic and/or supernatural interventions. It is for this reason that these pre-Socratics, and their heirs, the writers of the Hippocratic *Corpus* and Greek culture of the fifth century in general have been credited by some scholars as the originators of our modern scientific method.[8] Indeed so much has this been the case that some scholars have been moved to counter-balance this tradition by emphasising that the Greeks still retained an 'irrational' side.[9] In terms of the history of Western thought, these men who chose to study nature have been said to have 'invented' the idea of the "naturalness of natural phenomenon".[10]

Concerning the study of *phusis*, one must exercise caution. As Lloyd advises in *Methods and Problems of Greek Science*, it is a

7. Luce (1992) 18.
8. Cf. Jones (1972) vol. I xv "the matter is even more striking than the style. The spirit is truly scientific, in the modern and strictest sense of the word"; and xvii, xviii, "the doctrine of the Epidemic group is certainly not of the philosophic kind [but of the scientific]." Edelstein (1967) 12 ff., 401-439 balances this view.
9. Dodds (1951). See also Edelstein (1967) 401-439, and Lloyd (1979) 11, and (1991) 418.
10. Longrigg (1993) 26, 27 and Lloyd (1979) 11 and (1991) 418.

mistake to assume that there was a single concept of nature among the Greeks.[11] There were many and varying concepts coexisting, and these not always 'rational'. The ideas of the Ionians and later thinkers such as Plato, Aristotle and the authors of the medical corpus, did not supersede but rather co-existed with popular religions, mystery cults and other forms of explanations of the world.[12] We must not approach their writings through our own term 'nature' and automatically assume their study of *phusis* was equivalent to our science of physics.[13] Lloyd is also careful to point out that even among the *phusikoi* these principles were not agreed on by every great thinker. Edelstein, too, notes that

> Science was not yet an aggregate of opinions on which all scientists must and do agree.... For science as it was elaborated by the various Presocratic philosophers or scientists of the classical age really expressed their individual conviction, which was true in the opinion of its respective proponent and his pupils but of no validity for anyone else.[14]

For Lloyd, as regards the earliest Milesian philosophers, the actual written evidence of their thoughts about *phusis* is so fragmentary as not to bear the weight of investigation. Evidence from doxographical sources counts for little, since it may reflect as much the viewpoint of the later writer as the actual source. He prefers to concentrate on the more extensive writings of the medical corpus, Aristotle and Plato.[15]

If, then, we take these exceptional thinkers, as Lloyd and Edelstein suggest, on their own terms, what does 'phusis' and its study, mean? It means the effort to discover those principles which lie behind and explain natural phenomenon. And if we look carefully at the fragments we find a great irony. For, while distancing themselves from previous theological or magical

11. Lloyd (1991) 417.
12. Lloyd (1979) 10, Temkin (1995) 197.
13. Lloyd (1991) 417, 418.
14. Edelstein (1967) 435.
15. Lloyd (1991) 420.

explanations of the world and its phenomenon (a fact that has suggested to later scholars that they are our earliest scientists) the principles they discovered they nonetheless still considered to be divine.[16]

## Divine *Phusis*

In *Methods and Problems of Greek Science* Lloyd characterises their study as spanning the scientific, political and speculative, but also having 'metaphysical and philosophical assumptions' underlying it.[17] Longrigg concurs, emphasising that Thales and Anaximenes considered their first principles, their *arche*, to be divine, not in the sense of belonging to an anthropomorphic deity, but in that they were 'deathless and indestructible,' 'eternal and ageless'.[18] Though in seeming contrast, Empedocles and later Diogenes of Apollonia did name their primary elements as gods, or after gods, it may be that in all this their intention was merely to indicate that these principles were manifest in the gross physical as well as beyond the physical universe. But perhaps more importantly, the *phusikoi* managed to take the concept of divinity, which was previously associated with capriciousness and disturbance, and, by associating it with their *arche*, made it the manifestation of intelligible law,[19] which governs and gives order to the whole of nature, the whole of the universe, of life. Anaximander is credited by W.K.C. Guthrie with first describing this, using the word *kosmos*.[20] Phenomena are henceforth seen to be part of the grand regularity and constancy of nature which is intelligible, rather than subject to the whims of gods and demigods. Gregory Vlastos has observed that the presocratics transposed the "name and function of divinity into a realm conceived as rigorously rational order." [21] This new outlook has also been called the "spiritual discovery of the cosmos," and represents a

16. Lloyd (1979) 11, Edelstein (1967) 229: "the rational element in the medical art is divine."
17. Lloyd (1991) 418, 430.
18. Longrigg (1993) 31.
19. Ibid., 32. Longrigg is citing Vlastos in Allen and Furley (1975).
20. Guthrie (1962) vol. I 208, n.1.
21. Longrigg (1993) 32 quoting Jaeger, *Paideia*, I, fr. 158.

radical break with religious beliefs, the 'dividing line between religion and philosophy'.[22] They still used the concept of 'gods'—one of Thales' most cryptic fragments states 'all things are full of gods'—but made it the "name of a power (*dunamis*) which manifests itself in the operation, not the disturbance of intelligible law".[23] Perhaps this is why Guthrie points out that although shifting to the realm of the rational for their explanations, the thinkers were, even if unconsciously, still influenced by the prevailing milieu of recognising the existence of a realm beyond the material and physical.[24]

We know of the ideas of these early thinkers merely by the few fragments of the writings, often only recorded titles of works now lost. Besides these fragments of writings by early philosophers, we have for our knowledge of the early thinkers the more extensive, though second-hand, explanation of their thought in the writings of later philosophers. The writings of Aristotle, our authority for the doctrine of the Milesian philosophers, tell us that the first philosophers "thought the principles which were of the nature of matter were the only principles of all things. That of which all things that are consist, the first from which they come to be, the last into which they are resolved (the substance remaining, but changing in its modifications) this, they say, is the element (*stoiche*) and this the original principle or source (*arche*) of things and therefore they think nothing is either generated or destroyed, since this sort of entity is always conserved.... For there must be some entity—either one or more than one—from which all other things come to be, it being conserved. Yet they do not all agree as to the number and the nature of these principles."[25]

## The Stuff of Life

Among the varieties of explanations for these divine basic elements or *archai* of life, and of the universe we find the following. For the first, Thales, it was water, again, a concept not unconnected

22. Guthrie, ibid. He is quoting Jaeger, *Paideia*, I, fr. 158.
23. Vlastos cited in Longrigg (1993) 32.
24. Guthrie (1957) 11-12.
25. Sambursky (1963) 6, and Aristotle, *Metaphysics*, 98 3b.

with traditional belief, but now put to a new purpose. Water may have been chosen either because every food and seed contains water, or because as the God Ocean was considered the father of all things among the Ionians at that time, according to Aristotle. Or it may have been because water can be seen to change its nature and yet remain the same, like this first 'element', water can change form from solid, to liquid to vapour, and yet its substance remains the same. Anaximander, a second Milesian, posited a single *arche*, 'Non-Limited', *apeiron*, to point up the fact that it is beyond creation and destruction. According to Aristotle, for Anaximander

> there is some other non-limited substance from which all the heavens and the worlds contained in them came into being. The source from which existing things derive their existence is also that to which they return at their destruction, according to Necessity; for they give justice and make reparation to one another for their injustice according to the arrangement of Time.[26]

Anaximander felt this 'Non-Limited' was devoid of specific qualities itself, yet was still the substratum for all physical phenomena.[27] The Non-Limited was the ground of all being. Anaximander described the cyclical changes, the unending motions by which pairs of opposites separate off from the basic substratum of existence.[28] The fundamental pairs of opposites he identified are hot and cold, wet and dry.

For Heraclitus of Ephesus, air in the form of breath was associated with the intelligent life principle. He taught that men receive *logos* by breathing in [*logos* as thought conceived materially as breath, spirit].[29] Fire also he associated with *logos*. It was its material aspect, equated with soul-mind.[30]

For Anaximenes, the third of the Milesians, we find that as for Anaximander, the "first matter is one and unlimited." But, unlike Anaximander, he did not think that it is not specific, but that it is

26. Ibid., 8, from Simplicius, *Physics*, 24, 13 (Diels 12, A9). For a comparison of doxographical sources, see Kirk and Raven (1983) 107-108.
27. Ibid., 9.
28. Kirk and Raven (1983) 129, 119.
29. Ibid., 207. See also Onians (1994) 76-77, n. 9.
30. Guthrie (1962) vol. I 432, Kirk and Raven (1983) 199, fr. 30.

specific and like Heraclitus, associated it with air: *aer*.[31] *Aer* for Anaximenes differs in different things according to its rarity or density. Guthrie argues that 'by accounting for all quantitative differences of matter by different degrees of condensation and rarefaction of the one basic stuff, Anaximenes is already... demanding a quantitative explanation,' and that this constitutes a rational motive for the choice of air as *arche*. Guthrie thus seems to be arguing for a proto-scientific step here. But it is also possible that Anaximenes was motivated less to quantify natural phenomenon than by the conviction that there is no real separation between that universal 'ground' or 'substratum' and its individual manifestations. For, at the same time, as Guthrie himself suggests, Anaximenes was influenced by subconscious motives springing from the 'general climate of thought in which he and the other Milesian thinkers were living, and which they shared with their unphilosophical countrymen.' i.e. that the *assumption* that the "original source and fount of being (that is, for him, the air) had been in motion from all time and that this was what made its changes possible."[32]

For Anaximander, it was the 'Non-Limited', *apeiron*. For Anaximenes it was *aer*. But for each thinker there was a 'something' (a 'what is', *hen ti esti*, as the author of *Nature of Man* puts it) sought which would explain all phenomena we experience, much as Einstein sought a unified field theory twenty-five centuries later. According to J.V. Luce, though not Lloyd, with his reservations about the fragments, it is possible to infer from Thales' writings that he conceived of not only a vital fluid, water, but also a 'vital force' present in both animate and inanimate matter.[33] This term, 'vital force,' a term used by holistic practitioners today, could also be used for whatever the *arche* is conceived to be in explaining the basic source of nature by the different thinkers.

The interesting words used here are 'a sort of entity', 'first principle' and 'element', a 'something' for which different philosophers then offered different names, descriptions and

31. Kirk and Raven (1983) 144.
32. Guthrie (1962) vol. I 127.
33. Luce (1992) 21, 22.

explanations. It is further significant for our present subject that to these Milesian thinkers, including Thales and Anaximander, though not for the later Aristotle, there was "no opposition between an inert matter on the one hand and a force arousing it to motion on the other. The *arche* of the universe was not matter in that sense. It was eternal being, and because eternal and the *arche* of everything else, it was of necessity uncaused or else self-caused."[34]

Guthrie goes on to ask what to those of this time answered to this same description of 'self-caused'. He finds the answer to be *psuche*, which he translates as both 'soul' and 'life'. Thus, he says the *arche*, which for Anaximenes was *aer*, was 'eternal', *aidion*, 'immortal', *athanaton*, and therefore 'divine, *theion*.[35] Hence for these philosophers there was a divine vital force.

## Philosophers after the Milesians

From Miletus in the fifth century, the focus of philosophical activity seems to shift to southern Italy and somewhat later to Athens. We find Diogenes of Apollonia, also exalting the all-powerfulness of air, as the principle of life and thought. Diogenes wrote of air as the primal element from which all things are derived.

> Mankind and other living creatures live by means of air, through breathing it. And this is for them both soul (*psuche*) and intelligence (*phronein*)...And it seems to me that that which has intelligence is what men call air, and that all men are steered by this and it has power over all things. For this very thing seems to me to be a god...of all living creatures the soul is the same, air that is warmer than outside, in which we exist, but much cooler than that near the sun.[36]

We also have the writings and thought of Pythagoras, then of Alcmaeon and Empedocles, who were roughly contemporaneous. As the Diogenes fragment above shows, a certain shift of

34. Guthrie (1962) vol. I 128.
35. Ibid.
36. Kirk and Raven (1983) 434-435, Simplicius, fr.4, 5.

focus seems to have occurred. Eternal, primordial *archai* have been drawn down into the context of man and animals. The subject of interest is no longer just nature in general or external phenomena like earthquakes, storms and eclipses, but more specifically the 'nature of man'. For these later thinkers, the 'why and how' of the universe was connected with their curiosity about the nature of man and his relationship with the divine and also with the human body. In the Empedocles fragment 134.5, *kosmos* is associated with 'divine mind'. 'Mind alone', holy and beyond description, darting through the whole cosmos with swift thoughts, *alla phren hiere kai athesphatos epleto mounon phrontisi kosmon hapanta kataissousa thoesin.*[37]

Pythagoras held that all nature is in kinship, that life passes from one body to another (transmigration) and therefore we should abstain from eating animal flesh. A community of followers grew up around him, somewhat like a religious order. According to Guthrie, he greatly enriched and developed the concept first recorded by Anaximander that the world exhibits a comprehensible rational order. Like is known by like, and if we have any knowledge of the divine, it is not because of any sense organ but because we have in ourselves an essence of the divine element which recognises its self. The object of philosophy is to seek through it a better understanding of the structure of the divine *kosmos,* to realise and cultivate the divine element in oneself.[38] For Pythagoras, there were two *archai,* 'limit' and 'unlimited' but with these are equated odd and even numbers and from these are generated the material world.[39] According to Aristotle, Pythagoreans "supposed the elements of numbers to be the elements of all things and the whole heaven (*ton holon*) to be a *musical* scale (*harmonian*) and a number."[40] They also identified ten pairs of opposites (limit-unlimited, odd-even, one-plurality, male-female, right-left, light-darkness, square-oblong, at rest-moving, straight-crooked, good-bad].[41] From such ideas

37. Guthrie (1962) vol. I, 208-209, n 1. Kirk and Raven (1983) 350.
38. Guthrie, ibid 209-210.
39. Guthrie (1962) vol. I 246.
40. Aristotle, *Metaphysics*, 985b 23, Kirk and Raven (1983) 237.
41. Ibid. 238. Though the pairs named differ, this recalls the pairs of opposites in *Caraka* (Sharma and Dash, 1995, 422, Sūtrasthāna XXV, paragraph 36).

Pythagoras and his followers made advances in mathematics and the harmonics of music, but for our purposes here it is sufficient to note that his number theory is felt to be influential in the *Epidemics* which carefully note the progress of disease on odd and even days from its beginning. His views on the nature of man and the cosmos as divine, are also very influential in the thought of Plato, especially evident in the *Timaeus*.[42] The *Timaeus* also propounds a theory of health and disease similar to many of the ideas found in the Hippocratic *Corpus*.

Empedocles of Acragas lived between 492 and 432 B.C. Some traditions hold him to have been at one time a Pythagorean, and though he left the brotherhood, his thought is held to be similar to that of Pythagoras in many ways.[43] For him air was not a soul or source of beingness but one of the four self-existent 'root' elements, the others being fire, earth and water, from which all other things derive through the various minglings, or mixture, *krasis*, of these original four by the operation of *harmonia*. Empedocles used the term 'poros' for ducts or passages which exist in the skin and are involved in respiration.[44] They also make possible the 'mingling' or *krasis*, between the four 'root elements' brought about by Love. Air, for him the word used now is *pneuma*, was one of the four root elements, but also in its aspect as breath it was associated with the cosmic life principle.[45]

Empedocles was also interested in digestion and nutrition and worked out a theory of tissue nutrition from food via blood and the actions of the liver. According to Longrigg, this subsequently became the most widely accepted view of digestion in European medicine until the 17th century.[46] Blood too, he believed, was linked to respiration and thought, perhaps because

42. Guthrie (1962) vol. I 214.
43. Ibid., 208-209 n. 2.
44. Furley and Wilkie (1984) 3-5.
45. Ibid., 6. For Empedocles, "respiration was not purely physiological theory in any sense. Breath was either identical with or closely related to one of the four cosmic elements that formed the basic of his whole picture." Elements are divine Kirk and Raven (1983) 337, fr. 59.
46. Longrigg (1993) 74-75.

he believed blood, or the blood vessels at any rate, contained air. Thus for him the seat of thought is the heart.[47] He was a remarkable person, boasting he could bring back from Hades the strength of a man who had died. He mentions that drugs can defend man against illness and old age and that he can cure by the 'word of healing'.[48]

Alcmaeon was a physician from Croton in Italy which already had a reputation for having an excellent medical tradition.[49] He was very interested in physiology and sensation, carrying out dissections of the eye, developing his explanation of how the eye sees (a combination of the fire in it and the watery membrane covering). He was aware of the tissues which connect the brain to the eye and called these pores, 'poros'. Explaining hearing, he wrote of the existence of a void, *kenon*, which can be identified with air,[50] through which the sound echoes in the ear. He also described the arteries as containing air or *pneuma*, and the veins blood. He viewed the body as composed of *dunameis* or physical powers which when in equilibrium, *isonomia*, provide health but when separated and out of equilibrium, *monarchia*, produce disease.[51]

Another influential thinker about whom we have less evidence was Philistion. According to Galen (*De usu respirationis1*) he held that respiration is for the sake of preservation of innate heat. In *Anonymus Londinensis* (XX, 42-47) it is reported he believed that "when the whole body breathes well and breath passes through unhindered, health is the result."[52]

A final influential early thinker whose ideas would have been known to the writers of the Hippocratic *Corpus* was Democritus. He is known to have emphasised sound regimen (diet), and prevention before cure and felt that people frequently destroy their own health through ignorance and intemperance.[53] Democritus postulated an atomic theory: the basic particles of

47. Furley and Wilkie (1984) 6.
48. Longrigg (1993) 69, Kirk and Raven (1983) 354-355.
49. Guthrie (1962) vol. I 346.
50. Ibid., 349-350.
51. Ibid., 345, Longrigg (1993) 63.
52. Jones (1947) 81 (passage XX.24).
53. Longrigg (1993) 67.

the universe were atoms which moved about and came together into substances and forms. These atoms also make up the soul, so the soul had a material basis. He believed that the vehicle of life was *pneuma*, transmitted by way of semen.[54]

From this account we see that the writings of these early fifth century thinkers use their ideas of the nature of cosmic and divine principles to explain bodily processes, concepts which find echos in the later medical writers: for example, the physiology of perception, the seat of the intellect, the cause of sleep, the first parts of the body to develop from the embryo, the nature of semen, reproduction and sex differences, the nature of nutrition, and respiration, innate heat, and freely flowing breath as a health giving, and maintaining function.[55]

## Change and Continuity

Although we find a kind of revolution has occurred in the way man conceives of himself and his relationship to nature and to the divine, and that the new spirit is one of rational thought about the origins of life, at the same time many of the words used to describe this new position are ones that continue to carry the weight of their previous meanings and thus a measure of continuity between the old and new is maintained. The work of R.H. Onians has shown that certain concepts found in these philosophers and in the medical works do have links to those of the archaic period and the poems of Homer, Hesiod and the poets. For example, he has traced the idea that the seat of thought and feeling is located in or near the heart, and that breathing is connected with life and intelligence which flows into the area of the lungs and thymus from these writers into those of later periods.[56] The presocratics or *phusikoi*, the philosophers of nature, while attributing phenomena to the rational order of natural events, themselves did not abandon a sense of a divine something beyond the physical world or reject its existence, although some subsequent thinkers, the sophists seem to have. (Plato was partly

54. Ibid., 68.
55. Most of these are summarised by Longrigg (1993) 54-57.
56. Onians (1994) 23-43.

concerned to re-establish the place of an eternal, hence divine, moral order in the face of the merely relativist positions of the sophists.) Even the momentous mathematical advances of the Pythagoreans came within a spiritual discipline in which numbers were seen as the primary elements of a universe that was harmonious. The Pythagoreans' way of life was as much concerned with truth and justice as music and numbers. Indeed the two were inextricably linked.[57]

Still continuing alongside this shift in outlook and maintained by many people of all classes and education were the previous traditional Homeric concepts. Although there was no dominating monotheistic religion or priestly class, various religious practices, festivals and rituals were still observed. As for concerns about health and disease, one might say that people now had a choice, while some continued to attribute disease to the actions of a god or possession by a demon others chose to view it in a rational light, while maintaining a sense of the involvement of ultimate supra-rational forces. In society, though many people consulted the itinerant or state-appointed and funded physicians, whether slave or free professionals, many resorted to sellers of charms (charlatans according to the author of *The Sacred Disease*), or to the temple physicians of Asclepius and other healing deities to recover their health.[58] All these different approaches and concepts seemed able to co-exist. There were and continued to be many competing currents of thought and practice with no one dominating exclusively, "a pagan society that demanded respect for the gods but left much freedom for speculation about the divine...and moreover secular."[59]

## Philosophy and Medicine

We find, then, that in spite of the many examples of rational and scientific observation in the Hippocratic *Corpus*, the writers maintained

57. Guthrie (1962) vol. I 213 e.g. the number four symbolised the moral quality of justice.
58. For a discussion of the mutual influences between temple physicians and Hippocratic ones, see Edelstein (1967) 226, 244-246.
59. Temkin (1995) 197.

and were heirs of this congenial blend of acute observation and awareness of the divine in physical phenomena. The author of *The Sacred Disease* did object to explanations of disease and cure based on demonic possession, or individual supernatural occurrences, but did not repudiate the divine as such. Others allowed for prayers and believed that temple medicine could be useful.[60] While the author of *Ancient Medicine* argued against such philosophical concepts as "heat, cold, moisture and dryness" and against the philosopher Empedocles in particular, he nevertheless made use of the ideas of *krasis*/mingling and of digestion, which itself associates with heat.[61] The author of *Nature of Man* argued the point of view of one vein of philosophy, that of the pluralists, against that of another, the monists.[62] In other works, perhaps written with different purposes and audiences in mind, there is more of the philosophical side.[63]

Therefore, in the works of the collection, where there is no hint or mention of a divine principle, this would not seem to be a repudiation of the divinity of the cosmos but due to the strictly practical nature of the work. For physicians, the focus would naturally be more practical. They were interested in what worked, what got results. Theories were useful to the extent that they explained results achieved, leading to new fields of fruitful knowledge. Perhaps their attitude can best be summed up by the writer of *The Sacred Disease:* all diseases are both natural and divine.

Within such an understanding of the cosmic context in which human life and health unfold, the physicians worked. Many of

---

60. Edelstein (1967) 244-246. Temkin (1995) 85, 187-188. *Regimen*, Book IV.
61. *Ancient Medicine*, III, XIV. In XX, he seems to be arguing less that philosophy is irrelevant to medicine than that "knowledge of what man is, by what causes he is made and similar points, can best be learned by medicine itself *properly comprehended*" [emphasis mine]. In other words physicians were philosophers too. This compares with *Caraka* Sūtrasthāna I, 1-17, XXV 1-29; Śārīrasthāna I (Sharma and Dash 1994, vol. I 3-19; 415- 419; vol II 310 ff), which explicitly includes a philosophical element as context for its approach.
62. *Nature of Man*, II Jones (1979) xxviii.
63. For example, *Nutriment* reflects Hereaclitus while *Regimen* I, IV reflects the view that all of nature is divine and that "there is life in the things of the other world, as well as in those of this." Jones (1972) 337.

the views of these early physicians have resonances for a holistic practitioner of today. The recognition of an intelligible spiritual or divine element in man and in the cosmos at large, that the human organism includes mind and soul as well as body, that breath forms the link between these three, was part and parcel of the world view of the Hippocratic physicians. The concept that optimum health is a dynamic balance or harmony between different aspects including elemental energies, such as fire, water, air, and earth, is part of the holistic approach of many practitioners today. These concepts have not needed importation from 'Eastern philosophies'. Finally there is today a confirmation of that ancient attitude that,

> For these people, the natural world was not an object suitable [just] for experience, analysis and exploitation. It was not an object at all. It was alive with certain mysteries and powerful forces, and man's life still possessed a richness and a dignity which came from his sense of participation in the movement of these forces.[64]

Longrigg, Jones, and Lloyd among others have regretted the close connection between philosophy and medicine summarised above, or been keen to point out the differences between them as if the non-philosophical are the aspects of value while the others are not.[65] They tend to dismiss the 'schematic', theoretical side of ancient medicine, and emphasise its attention to hard facts. However, for a holistic practitioner this aspect is a very positive one, and for an important reason. It prevents medicine from becoming merely the understanding and treatment of disease, from reducing illness to the exclusively material level. It allows it to retain the understanding that treatment of illness affects the whole human being. Moreover, as Hans Seyle points out, "it is not

---

64. Guthrie (1962) vol. I 212. He is quoting Phillip Sherrard, *The Magic Threshing Floor*, 128. Guthrie feels this principle applies to Pythagorean thought particularly.
65. Jones (1981) vol. II, xxxix, Longrigg (1993) 69, 82, 99, Lloyd (1978) 44-45, 49. Lloyd does point out the fruitfulness as well as the limitations of the medical writers' use of analogies.

enough to recognise facts, we must also try to formulate ideas about the way the body behaves in health and disease. Only such theoretic concepts can guide us logically to new facts."[66]

## The Hippocratic Physician and His Society

Having briefly examined the relationship between philosophy and the Hippocratic writings, we can now consider the social context in which the physicians practised. We have seen that their philosophy was not abstract, but eminently practical and interwoven with daily life. Perhaps this explains the difference in explanations of disease in the *Corpus*: each writer used that explanation which seemed best to fit the facts of his experience. While acknowledging that some occurrences were beyond their explanations or skills to influence, where they could, they would relieve suffering by their *techne*, or craft of medicine. Treatises such as *The Art* and *Prognostikon*, show physicians were carefully taught to distinguish those diseases, or cases, which were considered to be curable.

For the most part the descriptions of disease in the *Corpus* are of acute ailments: fevers, infections and inflammations (e.g. nephritis, tuberculosis), wounds, sprains and fractures. Other conditions, perhaps chronic ones or ones which could not be treated by natural means, they would not consider to come within their realm of skills, and left to prayer, or the divine in general, but not to a specific deity. Deciding what they could treat was part of prognostics.[67] But the physician was equally interested in preventing disease and the maintenance of a healthy life for the individual and there is much attention in the *Corpus* given to this.[68]

Upon what type of people were they practising these skills? Greek society since about the seventh century B.C. was organised around the city-state, a town with its surrounding countryside. Within the society there were the free, adult male *politai*, whose legitimacy was based on membership in a clan group. Such men were to a large extent self-sufficient land and property owners,

---

66. Seyle (1984) 168.
67. *Prognostikon, The Art* VIII. See also Temkin (1991) 187-188.
68. For example, *Regimen I*, III; *Ancient Medicine* and *Regimen in Health*.

who participated in the public affairs of the state to different degrees in different cities, with degrees of status also based on age, wealth and noble lineage. Those wealthy enough to realise some leisure might become philosophers, artists or athletes, even gentlemen physicians. A *metoikos* was a free resident alien, with no political rights. The unfree *douloi* were males and females in servitude of various types. Free women enjoyed no political rights, and the desired norm was marriage and family. Some of noble lineage could be priestesses. *Hetairai* were women, slave, free or foreign, who were paid for sexual favours. Some women, for example Sappho, became poets, others midwives. Unless a priestess, midwife, *hetairai*, or slave, a woman was likely to be her husband's helpmate in the running of the household *oikos*. We find examples of such people mentioned as cases in the *Corpus*. Sometimes the physician was attending those ill with serious, acute ailments. (*Epidemics, Regimen in Acute Diseases*). Sometimes he was advising on the best way to maintain health (*Regimen I*). Unlike other cultures of the time, in Greece the ideas of democracy and equality before the law had been developing, especially in Athens, with every free man (though not women) allowed to vote and participate in public debates and political decisions. An individual's accomplishments, whether as athlete, sculptor or philosopher, were valued so that already a certain tension had developed between society and the individual. Outside of Athens too, Greeks thought of themselves as freemen, not subject to either kings or priests. There was both a sense of local identity and exposure to external influences through trade, wars and diplomatic links with Egypt, Palestine, the Persian empire and beyond, even to India.

Within such a society physicians worked. They, or at least those whose writings we still have, considered their work an art or craft: a *techne* based on learned skills and knowledge gained by observation and reason beyond common sense.[69] They worked for fees. Like the modern complementary practitioner, they sometimes felt the need to defend their profession against

69. An excellent discussion of this topic is found in Edelstein (1967) 102 ff.

the criticism that it was useless, or that people often got well by themselves, or through the use of charms or temple medicine. This situation is reflected in such treatises as *The Art, The Sacred Disease*. Some followed the medical profession as merely a means of earning a living. Others saw it as part of a wider philosophical life, or even as a holy vocation, as is shown in such works as *Decorum*, and *The Oath*. The latter work Edelstein has argued convincingly is connected to the Pythagorean school.[70] To learn their art students may have apprenticed themselves to a working physician, or have studied at a famous 'school' under an acknowledged master-teacher such as Hippocrates, a member of the Asclepiad. This professionally prestigious clan, whose patron was the hero–god Asclepius, was one in which medicine had been practised and handed down for generations. Eventually it may have opened its doors to outsiders.[71]

The physician seems to have occupied a rather special, if precarious and ambivalent place in society. There were no official courses of training or licensing of physicians. Each had to earn esteem by merit, sometimes aided by skills of rhetoric or persuasion. On the one hand he was just another healer in competition with rhizomatists (itinerant herb or root sellers who also offered treatments or advice), charm sellers, midwives, practitioners of healing cults, and other doctors, just like any artisan or seller of skills—as the word *techne* can imply. Edelstein finds that for the patient, the physician was not the educated authority figure of today's medical science but "a craftsman who must prove he knows his business [and whose] authority must be established."[72] His attitude toward his treatment is "shaped by conscious consideration of the person of the patient."[73] On the other hand, because of these skills and rational knowledge relating to healing (and the Greeks rated health very highly)[74] physicians were often highly valued. Even in the sixth century some cities appointed physicians for the general populace to consult.[75]

70. Ibid., 9-63 See also Sigerist (1987) 303.
71. Sigerist (1987) 300, Edelstein (1967) 40-41, Jones (1972) vol. I xlv.
72. Edelstein (1967) 88.
73. Ibid., 99.
74. Sigerist (1987) 299.
75. Ibid., 311. See also Lloyd's introduction to *Hippocratic Writings* (1978) 13, 15.

Or they could be among the company of leisured philosophers, as was Eryximachus who attended the famous dinner party described by Plato in *The Symposium.* While some might have remained in one place, many were itinerant, travelling from place to place and setting up their surgeries temporarily in the market place, or attending the more well-off in their homes. *Airs, Waters, and Places,* especially testifies to the skills of observation needed by an itinerant Hippocratic physician, while *The Physician,* and *Surgery* offer descriptions of how to set up the consulting room. As in many non-Western countries today, the relatives, friends or merely interested passers-by, even other doctors, might be present at such a consultation, each offering his or her own ideas if the physician seemed unsure.

Before turning our attention to the system to be compared, Ayurveda, it should be noted that the context of ancient medical writings is an interesting and relevant one for today's practitioner of holistic, complementary medicine. Like the Hippocratic physician, today's practitioner is as yet unregulated by legal statute. She (or he) must defend and justify the efficacy of her therapy by rational argument, and she is in competition with several other forms of healing, ostensibly non-rational, such as the use of gemstones (equivalent to ancient amulets) and 'spiritual healing' (to which physicians are beginning to refer patients in intractable cases, not unlike the relationship between the Hippocratic doctor and the healing cults). Like the Hippocratic physician, but unlike the prevailing view of the medical science physician, she acknowledges the existence of a divine or at least non-material life-force in nature, which affects the patient, the illness and its outcome. Her skills are grounded in working with this life-force to foster the healing process rather than dictating a cure to the body.

Returning to the situation in the fifth and sixth centuries B.C., we find that until recently their "revolution of wisdom" was believed to be peculiar to Western culture and that the start of scientific methods were attributed to Greece in this period. While we have seen that a change did occur, it was not unique to the West and as our examination of the *Corpus* shows, it could equally be argued that the foundations of holistic medicine were also established at this time. A similar turning point toward rational thought and philosophy occurred in the same centuries both in China and in India when rational explanations of human experience were also sought and found.[76] We will now turn to that era in ancient India and place the Ayurvedic treatise *Caraka-Saṃhitā* within its context.

## *CARAKA-SAṂHITĀ* IN CONTEXT

The principal text of Āyurveda used in this thesis for comparison purposes with the Hippocratic *Corpus* is the *Caraka-Saṃhitā*. *Caraka* (pronounced 'charaka') is one of three texts which form the written foundations of Āyurveda. The other two are *Suśruta-Saṃhitā* and *Bheda-Saṃhitā*. *Suśruta* is considered to cover the same material as *Caraka* but in more condensed form and with additional writings on surgery.[77] *Bheda Saṃhitā* has come down to us only in a fragmented and corrupted form.

*Saṃhitā* means compendium or compilation and this seems a fitting description of the text, as it includes different ideas and viewpoints on medicine as well as philosophical, religious and magico-religious elements. The translation of the text used for this investigation is that of R.K. Sharma and Bhagwan Dash. This translation includes a commentary by the 11th century author Cakrapāṇidatta, considered to be very authoritative. Cakrapāṇidatta has arranged the sequence of *sthānas* (sections), co-ordinated scattered facts and provided grammatical, philosophical and syntactic interpretation of difficult or technical terms used. He also provides colloquial and vernacular names of drugs and foods mentioned.[78]

Julius Jolly records that, according to Indian tradition and the *Caraka Saṃhitā* text, the 'knowledge (*veda*) of long life (*āyu*)' is received ultimately from Brahman, in Vedic religion the eternal soul and cause of the universe. From Brahman the knowledge or science of life is traced through Prajāpati, an aspect of Brahman as master of created things, through the twin gods

76. Woodcock (1989) 233, 241-244.
77. Filliozat (1964) 26.
78. Sharma and Dash (1995), vol. I xxxix, xl, xli.

Āświns, to the gods of human form, such as Indra, the god of warriors, but also god of Nature. Indra exposed the Āyurveda to the human Bharadvāja. Punarvasu, son of Atri (Ātreya) received the knowledge from Bharadvāja and transmitted it to six disciples out of the fifty *ṛṣis* (sages) who surrounded him. One of these, Agniveśa, composed a text of the knowledge, as then did the other five and, with the blessing of Ātreya, these six books became authoritative. The work is thus said to be composed by Agniveśa and revised by Caraka. Parts of the text have been revised or re-edited by a later writer, Dṛḍhabala, who lived before AD 300.[79] According to its own tradition then, the work is traced to mythical figures, gods, and to legendary humans (*ṛṣis*) who received the knowledge (the tradition seems to suggest) through mystical revelation.

Filliozat believes that "most probably the author who has created the legend of the transmission of Āyurveda, as found in the *Caraka Saṃhitā*, has found it proper to suppose that the pupil of Bharadvāja had been the same personage as one who had been described by tradition."[80] That there were one or more Ātreyas traditionally famed as medical doctors is possible, but there is no evidence that the legends of the origins of Āyurveda contain any real historical souvenir.[81] It is impossible also to say that the author is an historical figure and to date the works by his lifetime. Only textual study can resolve this.[82] However, besides its magico-religious material, the text does contain much rational and scientific material and this doctrine is derived from Brāhmaṇic speculations about the world.[83]

Zysk believes that Chattopadhyaya is probably right when he argues that *Caraka Saṃhitā*, in its original form was not the

---

79. Jolly (1994) 11, 15, and Sharma and Dash (1995) xxxix. Other classical texts of Āyurveda, e.g. *Suśruta* and *Bheda*, record variant traditions of transmission.
80. Filliozat (1964) 9.
81. Ibid., 9-11. He goes on to note that a historical figure, preserved in Buddhist text, is the doctor Ātreya, of Takṣasila (Taxila) the Buddhist university centre; the same site as that later visited by Alexander. He appears in the stories of Jīvaka, doctor to the king Bimbisara and also to the Buddha. However, this is unlikely to be the same person, as *Caraka* shows Ātreya teaching in on the Ganges and not in Taxila.
82. Ibid., 31.
83. Ibid., 31.

work of one person but the "compilation of medical knowledge of ancient roving physicians [Chattopadhyaya] [because] the treatise itself refers to different approaches to medicine and mentions numerous medical traditions...[the] word *caraka* means a wanderer or ascetic and aptly fits members of *sramaṇa* groups, the repositories of ancient medical lore. *Caraka* might also have been the name of a certain *sramaṇa*-physician who was court physician to the Kushana king, Kanishka, and may have participated in editing and compiling an already existing body of medical lore, but the evidence thus far marshalled does not confirm this."[84]

## ORGANISATION AND CONTENT

The text of *Caraka* comprises 120 chapters divided into eight sections or *sthānas:*

> *Sūtrasthāna* discusses pharmacology, food, diet, some disease and treatments, physicians, quacks and some philosophic topics.
> *Nidānasthāna* discusses the causes of eight main diseases.
> *Vimānasthāna* discusses taste, nourishment, pathology and medical studies.
> *Śārīrasthāna* discusses the fundamental principles of the universe along philosophic lines—the origin of mankind—and thus includes embryology and anatomy.
> *Indriyasthāna* discusses diagnosis and prognosis.
> *Cikitsāsthāna* discusses specific therapies.
> *Kalpasthāna* discusses pharmacy.
> *Siddhasthāna* has further discussion on therapy.[85]

Within this organisation we find that in fact many topics are discussed in several other sections, the siddhisthāna overlapping each other in content. This characteristic supports the view that it is a compilation of different strands of healing traditions.

The text is written in both prose and verse, some chapters being exclusively verse except for a prose beginning and colophon. Some chapters are statements by the Teacher (Agniveśa)

84. Zysk (1991) 33.
85. Wujastyk (1998) 41.

giving instructions; some are based on enquiries by the student in dialogue form with the teacher; some are statements of the Redactor, Caraka; and others are in the form of discussions among individual physicians engaged in a seminar. In his introduction, R.K. Sharma notes that some irrelevant statements have been interpolated into the texts, along with several contradictory statements.[86]

Although many contemporary teachers and practitioners of Āyurveda like to represent it as being about 4,000 to 5,000 years old,[87] in terms of textual sources this is indeed not the case. It is, however, true that many of the concepts found in Āyurveda are traceable to the four ancient *Vedas* of that period, the *Ṛgveda*, the *Sāmaveda*, the *Atharvaveda* and the *Yajurveda*. The *Vedas* are the epic hymns of the Āryan peoples about gods, demons, and heroes. Many of these hymns contain not only descriptions of healing gods and heroes, but mention specific healing plants, and give healing incantations. In addition, as Jean Filliozat has shown, concepts found in the classical texts like *Caraka*, such as *vāyu/prāṇa*, as well as certain diseases, and points of anatomy, are traceable to the Vedas.[88] More specifically, Āyurveda traces its roots to the *Atharvaveda*. This *veda* differs from the others in that it contains more material concerning disease and gives ways of ridding a person from disease using magico-religious means, such as incantations, amulets, prayers and sacrifices.

Only in this sense the statement about the ancient origins may be true. As a system of medicine, Āyurveda can be said to emerge only in the sixth to fifth centuries B.C. and its extant texts even later. The exact date of the composition is unknown; the earliest version is thought to date from about the third or second centuries B.C.[89] Our extant text is thought to date from the second century A.D.[90] In this text are found the magico-religious or ritualistic elements, but also a philosophical element and a clear rational system of medicine practised by trained physicians.

86. Sharma and Dash (1995), Vol.I xxxiv.
87. Zysk (1991) 117-118 and lecture at the Wellcome Institute, London, September 1996.
88. Filliozat (1964) Chapters 3, 4, 5.
89. Wujastyk (1998) 40.
90. Zysk (1991) 33.

While the extant text of *Caraka* is not as old as that of the Hippocratic treatises, the rational elements within it are now known to date from at least the sixth century B.C.

In *Caraka* it is stated that the work is a redaction of an earlier medical treatise by Agniveśa. The knowledge and practice contained in it is now thought to be a compilation of much older material and to derive from the sixth and fifth centuries B.C. Dr. Kenneth Zysk in his book *Asceticism and Healing in Ancient India*, and Debiprasad Chattopadhyaya in Science and *Society in Ancient India*, persuasively argue this case. They have looked at the earliest Buddhist texts, the *Pāli* cannon whose contents date from the time of the Buddha (fifth century B.C.), and at the practices and ideas of other ascetics, such as Mahavira (the founder of the Jains). These, like the Buddha, stood outside conventional brahmin-dominated society, wandering the jungles and gathering for debates during the rainy season.[91] Zysk and Chattopadhyaya have noted the great attention given to medicine by the Buddha, in contrast to its ostracism by the brahmins. They note also that much of the medical material in the *Pāli* is very similar to the theory and practice of Āyurveda as found in *Caraka* and *Suśruta*, both as to *materia medica* and therapeutic procedures. But the *Pāli* also contains magico-religious elements. Interestingly these elements are separated and are given their own section in Caraka under the classification for diseases which require recourse to the divine, i.e., for which no rational approach is effective or perhaps possible. Zysk argues that the irrational elements are preserved remnants of healing originating in Vedic times, since similar ones appear in the Atharvaveda.[92] He cites the treatment for morbid pallor or jaundice as evidence of rational Medicine:

> A certain monk suffered form morbid pallor or jaundice (*pāṇḍuroga*), for which he was given a solution of urine and yellow myrobalan to drink (*mutthaharitakam payetum*). Buddhaghosa explains that the treatment consisted of yellow myrobalan mixed with cow's urine.

91. Ibid., 21-27 and Chattopadhyaya (1979) 270-306.
92. Ibid., 32.

> In early medical treatises an entire chapter is devoted to the symptoms and treatment of morbid pallor... Both *Caraka* and *Suśruta* agree that the first and most important treatment for *pāṇḍuroga*, is the administration of a drug that evacuates the patient. Two principal remedies for accomplishing this are outlined: those using clarified butter as a base and those using the urine of cows or buffaloes as a base....
>
> The means of treating morbid pallor mentioned in Buddhist monastic medicine has correspondence in the two early medical treatises, illustrating a correspondence in medical doctrine and pointing to a common source for the medical traditions of *Caraka* and *Suśruta* as well as that of the early Buddhists.[93]

Other such correspondences which Zysk finds between the diagnosis and treatment of Buddhist monks and those in *Caraka* and *Suśruta* include: large sores, nonhuman disease, eye disease, head irritated by heat, affliction of wind [vāta], wind in the joints, split open feet, swellings, snakebite, effects of harmful drink, corruption of skin, defective digestion, body filled with 'peccant humours', wind in the abdomen, burning in the body, and rectal fistula.[94]

Like Zysk, Chattopadhyaya emphasises the interrelationship between the development of natural philosophy (from the eighth to sixth centuries B.C.) and the development of medicine. This development is recorded in the *Upaniṣads* (700-500 B.C.) whose subject is a philosophical enquiry into the nature of the universe and human consciousness. First, Chattopadhyaya feels that while the philosophers of the *Upaniṣads* were originally interested in direct knowledge of nature and the nature of man, due to the force of Brāhmaṇical mores this interest turned from being the

> knowledge of the object to the knowledge of the subject itself—the bare ego or pure self... and extreme inversion...

93. Ibid., 106-107.
94. Ibid., 84-116.

> the immediate result of which is the lofty contempt for nature or the material world.[95]

He points out that unlike the Vedic scriptures, there is little interest in medicine in the *Upaniṣads*. Chattopadhyaya then passes to the *Pāli* canon for its rational therapeutics *yukti-vyapasraya bheṣaja*. He concludes that sometime before the Buddha – i.e., not much later that the *Upaniṣads* – Indian medicine takes the prodigious step from magico – religious to rational.[96] According to Chattopadhyaya, the *Upaniṣads* themselves refer to groups of roving ascetics, "motley heretics united by their common antipathy for the scripture or Vedas"[97] and who include "logicians, denying soul on the strength of observation and reasoning...[and] physicians".[98] The *Upaniṣads*, he believes may be prejudiced when they describe these as practising only magico-religious healings, and suggests that perhaps the writers of the *Upaniṣads* did not bother to find out what the heretics were doing. In any case medicine "belongs to the ideological world of heretics".[99]

However, Chattopadhyaya argues that one *Upaniṣad*, the *Chāndogya* VII, does describe a philosopher, Uddālaka Aruṇi, who is more interested in natural phenomena than introspection, and disagrees with the prevailing view that everything comes into being from non-being, or void. 'In the beginning this world was just being – *sat*, one only without a second.' From this evolve three material elements, fire, water and food. Chattopadhyaya believes this materialist viewpoint is very like the slightly later philosophy of Sāṃkhya, and it is important to note that it is

95. Chattopadhyaya (1979) 280-281. This is very reminiscent of criticism made of Plato's thought and Western mysticism in general, as Chattopadhyaya himself notes on p. 28 ff. Also it must be remembered that the author is intent on showing that ancient medicine was originally exclusively material and rational, and would have gone on to develop along scientific lines but for the interference of the counter ideology of the brahmin caste. Any religious or philosophical content in the text is an attempt to mollify or conform to later more powerful religious norms, according to Chattopadhyaya. His position is not unlike that of Longrigg, Lloyd and Jones with respect to Greek medicine, see note 69 above.
96. Ibid., 341.
97. Ibid., 288-289.
98. Ibid., 290.
99. Ibid., 289-290.

arrived at not through scripture or revelation but through rational observation and inference.[100]

Chattopadhyaya's further evidence for a pre-Buddhist source of rational medical therapeutics is the link between Uddālaka and one Saunaka, who is mentioned in both *Caraka* and the *Śatapatha Brāhmaṇa* as specializing in physiology and anatomy and living outside the stronghold of Upaniṣadic culture. (*Brāhmaṇa* are texts concerned to record and explain vedic sacrificial rituals.) The *Śatapatha* tells us that Uddālaka chose to be his pupil, "the philosopher submitting himself to the physiologist for acquiring knowledge". Saunaka was also the clan name of a group found in the *Atharvaveda*, the *veda* containing the most emphasis on healing diseases, i.e., medicine, which Āyurveda looks to as its source.[101] This point, however, is not well attested to by other scholars.

Finally, Chattopadhyaya, points out that one of the heretical thinkers was the Buddha, who, rather than being interested in the Vedic priests or the "world-denying pure soul which dominates the Upaniṣads", showed a keen interest in medicine for the well-being of the monks.[102]

Thus both Zysk and Chattopadhyaya conclude that among the wandering ascetics were many medical ascetics, and that information was empirically gathered and exchanged among these, gradually building an oral tradition of knowledge. A reference to these wandering ascetics is also found in the Jain canonical text, *Vyākhyāprajñapti*.[103] and the first written documentation of their knowledge is the Buddhist *Pāli* canon.

> During the centuries intervening between Vedic medicine and the absorption of Indian medicine into brāhmaṇic orthodoxy, the medical paradigm dramatically shifted from a magico-religious to an empirico-rational approach to healing. This transition occurred largely because of close associations between medicine and the heterodox ascetic

100. Ibid., 292, 294, 298, 300.
101. Ibid., 303, 306-307.
102. Ibid., 324.
103. Zysk (1991) 27. The text is Bhagavatī Sūtra 15.539, 658-69.

> traditions of ancient India. The shunned medical specialists, wandering the countryside, administering cures to all who required (and could pay for) them, and closely studying the world around them while exchanging valuable information with their fellow healers, understandably gravitated toward those sharing a similar alienation and outlook. These were orthodox mendicants and the heterodox wandering ascetics. Such persons abandoned society to seek liberation from the endless cycle of birth, death, and rebirth, and were quite indifferent to or even antagonistic to the brāhmaṇic orthodoxy of class and ritualism based on sacrifice to the gods of the Vedic pantheon.
>
> The heterodox ascetic movements in ancient India provided a social and philosophical orientation found among both the early Buddhists and the early medical theoreticians. The healers, like the ascetics, were seekers of knowledge and outcasts, shunned by the orthodox Hindus. They wandered about performing their cures and acquiring new medicine treatments. Eventually they become indistinguishable from the other *sramaṇa* with whom they were in close contact. The healers were not necessarily ascetics... but many ascetics might well have been physicians. A vast storehouse of medical knowledge developed among these sramaṇic physicians, supplying the Indian medical tradition with the precepts and practices of what has come to be known as *āyurveda.*[104]

As we shall see below, in the account of a Greek visitor to India, Megasthenes, further details are found about the activities and knowledge of these heterodox ascetics with regard to health and disease. These accounts, together with the early Buddhist medical traditions in the *Pāli* canon confirm the existence, from at least the fifth and fourth centuries B.C. of what Chattopadhyaya argues is the essence of Āyurveda: an empirical and very rational system of medical therapeutics.[105] For Megasthenes's description

104. Ibid., 26, 37.
105. Chattopadhyaya (1979) 84.

of the philosophical orientation and the rational therapeutics based on dietary regimen and external use of drugs used by the Indian doctor closely fits that of the *Caraka-Saṃhitā* and the earlier Buddhist *Pāli* canon.

## PHILOSOPHICAL BACKGROUND TO *CARAKA* AND EARLY INDIAN MEDICINE

As Filliozat has suggested the rational and material aspects of the text derive from that post-Vedic period in India, after about 600 B.C., when a new spirit of speculation about the origins of being, neither priestly nor mythological in nature, emerges. This spirit is found in such texts as those of the *Upaniṣads* and in the teachings of the Buddha and Mahavira. The brahmin priests continued the Vedic religion and practices and considered religious observance of sacrifices and rituals and acceptance of law as of the utmost importance.

The *Upaniṣads* inquire into the origins of the phenomenal world and of individual consciousness. Being written over many years, they form part of but also grow beyond the *Brāhmaṇa* or directories of and explanations for these sacrificial rituals.[106]

> In a seemingly childlike manner, like the early Greek cosmologists, they advanced now one thing and now another as an image of the primary material out of which the whole world is made... and again like the early Greek philosophers, they were always aware of the underlying unity of all being....[they are a] first recorded attempt at systematic philosophising to construe the world of experience as a rational whole.[107]

The *Upaniṣads* are heterogeneous in material and in composition and present a variety of answers to the question, "What is the world made of?", e.g. water, space and an even greater abstraction, Non-being (*a sad*), as well as Being (*sad*) and the Imperishable.[108]

Later the concept of Brahma overcomes and absorbs into itself all these other ideas of the world-ground. This idea itself is found in the *Vedas* as that power inherent in its hymns and

---

106. Hume (1921) 5.
107. Ibid., 1, 2.
108. Ibid., 6, 10, 11, 12.

prayers, but *Upaniṣads*' insight is to "take the world from its religious connection and infuse it with a philosophical connection".[109]

Brahma itself is variously equated with ether, life, god, breathing, understanding and bliss. It is also becomes the universal soul or ātman and the source of all existence. It exists in the individual human being also, manifested as 'a person's psychical activity with its seat in the sense and mental organs' and providing intelligence, truthfulness and steadfastness.[110] In the *Upaniṣad Chāndogya*, 7.1, it is said that everything is breath and finally that the whole world is spirit or *Ātman*.[111] Thus the *Upaniṣads* reveal the microcosm-macrocosm relationship between man and the external cosmos and the inner ground of being. Brahma, the unitary Reality is present in objective phenomena and in the self's activities. In the later *Upaniṣads*, the idea of the individual Self or soul/*ātman* is united with that of Brahma into an essential monism.[112]

## Sāṃkhya Philosophy

Also found in some of the *Upaniṣads* are elements of what emerges later as *Sāṃkhya* philosophy,[113] one of the schools of philosophy which developed in India. Its model of the nature of reality conceives of an outer physical world including mankind, and an inner consciousness and source of creation. This is the model found in the text of *Caraka*. '*Sāṃkhya*' means knowledge or true knowledge and signifies a path of knowledge or philosophical wisdom leading to realisation of the true nature of the self as the immortal, all pervasive infinite.[114] The scheme of *Sāṃkhya* found in *Caraka* is similar to but subtly different from classical *Sāṃkhya* as described in Isvarakrisna's *Sāṃkhya Kārikā*, a fourth century A.D. text.[115] The similar, if distinctive,

109. Ibid., 14, 15.
110. Ibid., 18.
111. Ibid., 20.
112. Ibid., 21, 33.
113. Ibid., 8.
114. Dasgupta (1932) 455.
115. The question has not been answered as to whether Caraka's representation is a proto-sāṃkhya or just different, according to Anne Glazier.

ideas of other philosophical schools, such as Vaiśeṣika and Nyāya, are also found in *Caraka*, though to a lesser extent.[116] The medical texts in fact contain perhaps one of the earliest and one of the largest amounts of material about the ideas of philosophical schools. The schools of philosophy that contributed concepts to the medical profession were themselves still in flux in the period that produced the final redaction of the early texts.[117]

According to the model presented in *Caraka*, (e.g. Sūtrasthāna I, and Śārīrasthāna I) existence is explained by twenty-five cosmic principles or *tattvas*: *puruṣa* or ultimate being (eternal and not subject to change); *prakṛti* or primordial nature (eternal but changeable, out of which the world is created); *mahat* or cosmic intelligence; *ahaṃkāra* or individual ego; *manas* or mind; five *tanmātras* or subtle elements; five *jñānendriyāṇi* or sense faculties (hearing, touching, seeing, tasting, smelling); five *karmendriyāṇi* faculties of action (speaking, grasping, walking, evacuation and procreation); five *mahābhūtas* the gross or 'great' elements (earth, water, fire, air and ether); and a faculty of thought for ordinary mental and intellectual activities, *buddhi*.

In the human body, the five *mahābhūtas* are manifested in three aspects as the biological *doṣas: vāta* (*ākāśa* or ether and air), *pitta* (fire and water), and *kapha* (water and earth). While governing such physiological processes as bodily heat, digestion, growth of flesh, circulation and movement, each of the dosas also governs the different mental attitudes and the emotions. (See Appendix.)

We notice that in seeking an explanation for the nature of the physical world, the thinkers also related this directly to certain physiological faculties in the human organism, for example the five senses and the ability to move. From this inclusion of a philosophical perspective on the human organism in the medical text, we learn that the art of the ancient ayurvedic

116. Meulenbeld, privately circulated papers: Seattle lectures, p.4. He states the schools were still in flux in the period that saw the final redaction of the classical medical treatises and that the concepts borrowed from the schools were adjusted to medical purposes.

117. Ibid. By contrast, Chattopadhyaya argues that Nyāya-Vaiśeṣika derives its concepts from medical traditions. See 135-136.

physicians was informed by the ideas of a philosophy which viewed man as a part of the greater wholeness of nature, *prakṛti*, deriving ultimately from a single source or first principle, *puruṣa*. That *Caraka* includes several distinct philosophical traditions suggests several possibilities. One is that several strands of tradition are found in the compilation; another is that the physicians felt it important to ground their rational physical therapeutics within a larger philosophical context. It suggests that some of the physicians might simultaneously have been philosophers themselves. It also suggests that they were willing to adapt different philosophical approaches to the practicalities and needs of their own profession. The philosophical models gave them a system within which to organise, process and put to use the information derived by them from their observations of foods, plants, climate and geography, human behaviour, health and disease.

## The Physician and his Society

At this time in Indian history, people were living in villages and towns, in independent kingdoms or small republics. The migration by Indo-European peoples to the north-west Indian sub-continent between 3000 and 1500 B.C. had established them as the uppermost members of society (*āryan*, Sanskrit for noble), and they were related through a clan structure. The previous indigenous population was relegated to the lowest level of the social order. The aryans themselves were divided into the *brahmin* caste, responsible for preserving the group's identity and purity through its religion, the *kṣatriyas* or the warrior nobility, and the *vaiśyas*, those engaged in material and commercial affairs, farming and trade.[118]

From the Vedic period we have hints of a change in the status of medical practitioners. Among the priestly group we find evidence of a certain denigration of the role of the physician in society. Religious law was codified in such works as the *Law of Manu*. Chattopadhyaya makes much of the few lines in this text where physicians are termed 'defiled'. The

118. Another group of these peoples migrated west into Greece. Jean Sedlar (1980) points out some similarities of their culture based on common roots.

*Maitri Upaniṣad* speaks of practitioners of poison removal as heretics unfit for heaven and warns kings against listening to them. However, it is quite possible that such strictures were mainly intended for *brahmin* caste members only for whom physical contact with non-*brahmin* castes was abhorrent, or for those intent exclusively on spiritual liberation. These strictures may have derived from the idea that the most important things in life were religious observance and acceptance of the *Law of karma*, on the one hand, or on the pre-eminence of the spiritual practice on the other. If so, they would not reflect a universal attitude. Nevertheless, as the most revered members of society, what *brahmins* thought carried considerable influence. A marked change or exception to this attitude is marked by the heterodox ascetics, particularly the Buddha, who positively encouraged the use of medicine and modelled some of his teachings on it, (as did Plato). At any rate, despite such injunctions of *brahmins* and the *Law of Manu*, physicians continued to develop and practise their art, and to be sought after by kings and other wealthy members of society, as well as ordinary people.[119]

A fascinating insight into certain aspects of ancient Indian society actually comes to us from Greeks who travelled there. These sources date from slightly later than the Hippocratic treatises and there is no intention to suggest here a cross fertilisation. Zysk has highlighted the fact that they do serve to corroborate the existence of the early ascetics and physicians. The geographer-historian Strabo (*c.* 64 B.C.-A.D. 21) records fourth century B.C. observations of these heterodox ascetics and physicians by two Greeks: Onesicritus, a cynic philosopher and historian travelling with Alexander's army into India, and Megasthenes, the historian of Seleucus, Alexander's successor as ruler of his eastern empire in 323 B.C. Their accounts help us to envisage the way of life of the early physicians and philosophers.

From Onesicritus's report we learn about Alexander's encounter with these same heterodox ascetics in the area of Taxila. Alexander sent Onesicritus to summon them to his presence.

---

119. For example, the some treatments prescribed in *Caraka* suggest the need for many servants to carry them out, yet there is also acknowledgement that physicians also attended the poor. Cikitsāsthāna 52-62.

Onesicritus says that he found 15 men who were in different postures,

> standing or sitting or lying naked and motionless till evening... The first he approached, Calanus, laughed at him and then bade him, if he wished to learn to take off his clothes, and lie down naked to hear his teachings. Mandanis, 'the oldest and wisest of the group rebuked Calanus for arrogance and spoke to Onesicritus, saying his king (Alexander) was the only philosopher in arms he ever saw.' Calanus later joined Alexander as he marched back to Greece, but became ill on the way and immolated himself on a pyre.[120]
>
> At all events, all he [Mandanis] said, according to Onesicritus, tended to this, that the best teaching is that which removes pleasure and pain from the soul and that pain and toil differ, for the former is inimical to man and the latter friendly, since man trains the body for toil in order that his opinions may be strengthened, whereby he may put a stop to dissensions and be ready to give good advice to all, both in public and in private...Mandanis inquired whether such doctrines were taught among the Greeks; and that when he answered that Pythagoras taught such doctrines and also bade people to abstain from meat, as did also Socrates and Diogenes [the Cynic]...Mandanis replied that he regarded the Greeks as sound-minded in general, but that they were wrong in one respect, in that they preferred custom to nature; for otherwise, Mandanis said, they would not be ashamed to go naked, like himself, and live on frugal fare; for he added, the best house is that which requires the least repairs...They [the naked philosophers] inquire into numerous natural phenomena, including prognostics, rains, droughts and diseases....[121]

---

120. Strabo, 63-64 Jones 109-113.

121. Strabo 65, Jones 113-115. There is the hint of a striking similarity between this view and that of some Greek philosophers and physicians but it seems to contrast with the view of the author of *Nature of Man* that if man were 'one' he would feel no pain. (c. II).

This report suggests that like both the presocratics and Socrates and his followers, the Indian ascetics were interested in the study of both nature and 'man', including learning about weather, climate, and disease, and that by acute observation of they believed one could make rational predictions about their behaviour. Although we must take into account that Onesicritus, being a Cynic, may have reported the teachings of the ascetics in a light which emphasised their similarity to that of his own school of thought, nonetheless the report does confirm the existence of these ascetics and the outlines of their teachings, establishing a link between them and the practitioners of medicine. Onesicritus may be a reliable a witness, for as reported his details about the meditation practices of the gymnetai are broadly similar to what we know of the practices of other ascetics, such as the founder of Jainism, Mahavira (sixth century B.C.).[122]

A short time later, Seleucus sent Megasthenes to the court of Chandragupta, who from his capital at Pataliputra (now Patna) had consolidated his rule over a large territory and had halted the advance of the Greeks to the east.[123]

> And with regard to the Garmanes [i.e. *sramaṇas/ascetics*], Megasthenes says that some, the most esteemed, are called Hylobii [forest-dwelling], who live in the forests, [existing] on leaves and wild fruits, [wearing] clothing of tree bark, without [indulging] in sexual intercourse and wine. [He says that] they associate with the ones who, through messengers, inquire about the causes [of things]; and who through those [Hylobii] serve and petition the divinity. And after the Hylobii [Megasthenes says that] the physicians come second in [so far as] honour; and [that they are] philosophers, as it were, concerning mankind, frugal, but not living off the land, who sustain themselves with rice and barley groats, all of

---

122. There is an artefact from the earlier Harappan civilization of the Indus Valley which shows a naked man in a standing position very like that of the body-abandonment (kāyotsarga) poses of early Jain ascetics (the jinas or liberated beings), one of whose sects (the digambaras or sky-clad) was committed to going completely naked, feeling that any possessions were a hindrance to liberation. See Wheeler (1966), 41 and notes for the Jain exhibition, Victoria and Albert Museum, February, 1996.

123. Wheeler (1950) 39-40 and (1966) 115.

> which, [he says], the one who is begged and who welcomes them in hospitality, supplies to them; and [he says that] they are able to bring about multiple offspring, male offspring and female offspring, through the art of preparing and using drugs; but they accomplish healing through grains for the most part, not through drugs; and of the drugs [he says that] the most highly esteemed are the ointments and the plasters; but the rest have much that is harmful. And [he says that] both the latter and the former (*iatrikoi* and *garmanes*) practice endurance, both actively and inactively, so that they can continue being fixed in one posture the whole day; and there are others who are prophetic, skilled in the use of incantations, and skilled in the words and customs associated with the 'departed', and who go begging through both villages and cities; on the other hand [there are] others who are more attractive than these and more urbane; but even they themselves do not refrain from the common rumours about Hades, insofar as it seems to [tend] toward piety and holiness. And [he says that] women as well as [men] study philosophy and with some of them, and the women also abstain from sex.[124]

In another section Strabo also reports:

> The *Pramnai* are philosophers opposed to the Brachmanes, and are contentious and fond of argument. They ridicule the Brachmanes who study physiology and astronomy as fools, as impostors. Some of them are called *Pramnai* of the mountains, others the *Gymnetai* [naked philosophers] and others again the *pramnai* of the city and *pramnai* of the country. Those of the mountains wear deer skins and carry wallets filled with roots and drugs professing to cure diseases by means of incantations, charms, and amulets. The Gymnetai, in accordance with their name, are naked, and live generally in the open air, practicing endurance, as I have already mentioned, for seven-and-thirty years. Women live in their society without sexual commerce.[125]

---

124. Quoted by Zysk (1991) 28 from Strabo's *Geographia* Book XV, 15.1. 60-61.
125. Jones (1949) 15.1. 70.

From these sources we gain a fascinating insight into the society. We learn that there was a variety among these ascetics, that they played a role in advising kings as well as ordinary folk and held an esteemed place in society. They advised on maintaining health and also helped using food, drugs and external applications as well as magico- religious means. Also some women at least were free to become ascetics.

This evidence supports what we find in the text of *Caraka* itself. The nature of some of the treatments seem to indicate it was a text for physicians who would be attending the higher members of society since some of the therapeutics prescribed can be quite complicated to prepare and time-consuming to apply. However, in other parts, perhaps those which represent earlier material, as highlighted by Zysk, procedures are simpler and more straightforward, like the ones prescribed in the *Pāli* canon. In *Caraka* physicians are enjoined to be of service to humanity: "A person who pursues medical profession just out of compassion for the living being and not for *artha* (wealth) or *kāma* (satisfaction of the worldly desires) excels all others...compassion for living creatures is the *dharma* (righteousness) *par excellence.* A physician who enters the medical profession keeping this ideal in view, accomplishes his objectives best and gets happiness *par excellence.*"[126]

## SIMILARITIES AND DIFFERENCES BETWEEN *CARAKA* AND THE HIPPOCRATIC *CORPUS*

The sixth century B.C. stands between the earliest archaic and Vedic periods of ancient Greece and India, respectively, and the period in which we find the earliest written records of a rational system of medicine, the fifth century, a time of profound change and development. During this time, from which flowed new approaches to health and disease, a shift occurred from a magico-religious orientation towards a rational and philosophical approach to understanding human life, at least on the part of a significant and influential section of each society.

We have seen that Āyurveda consists of both a philosophical

126. Sharma and Dash (1995) 69 Cikitāsthāna I verses 52-62.

element and a rational therapeutic system. In this it is similar to Hippocratic medicine. *Caraka* also includes remnants of an earlier magico-religious approach. We find none of this in the Hippocratic treatises, and in fact in some such things are ridiculed. However, an awareness of nature as divine is very marked in the treatises of the *Corpus*, so they cannot be said to be exclusively materialistic and scientific in our modern sense of these words.

In both Greek and Indian culture these philosophic and medical traditions show variety in their explanations about the origins of life and of disease and health in human beings. In neither is there, at this point, a single dominant model, yet underneath the diversity is the common theme that there is a spiritual source for life, however it is named or conceived, and that human life is a microcosm of the greater macrocosm of nature. Ultimately health and happiness are found in trying to live in harmony with the macrocosm.

It may also be noted that both Hippocratic medicine and Āyurveda co-existed with other forms of treatment, such as incantations and temple-based religious practices. Physicians were itinerant in each culture; they might be consulted by the wealthy and by royalty as well as by ordinary people.

In both cases there is an early and close association with other rational thinkers. We may note from the reports of Onesicritus and Megasthenes that the ancient Indian 'heterodox ascetics' (as Zysk calls them) acted as wise counsel to local people ('advice to all both, public and private'). They interested themselves in disease and the physicians among them healed mainly through grains rather than 'drugs' (i.e. herbs, metals, animal products) but used some drugs, mainly externally as plasters and ointments. They held knowledge about promoting healthy reproduction. This role and approach recalls the therapeutics of some of the Hippocratics, which relied mainly on dietary therapy. We find in Greece that philosophers such as Alcmaeon were interested in medical questions. Plato often uses the medical practice as an analogy to explain some of his ideas about love, about the nature of man and society.[127] Similarly in India, the Buddhist texts show an interest in rational medicine.

---

127. E.g. *Charmides 156b,c Phaedrus 270, Symposium* 186-188.

From the Greek account we also learn that the naked and forest-dwelling philosophers gathered for discussion and argument. One such congregation may well have been like that described in *Caraka*, in which learned physicians gather to debate the medical question of the different types of *rasa* or tastes.[128] This is somewhat similar to the experience of the Hippocratic physicians. It is known that some of the treatises were written in rhetorical style, that is to argue and defend a certain view or practice, indicating that they were intended to be spoken or read in public debates. The evidence in *Caraka* and Strabo's account not only suggests that different strands of tradition may be woven into *Caraka*, but reveals that freedom of argument and debate was not unique to early Western thinking, as has been suggested by some scholars.[129]

The status of the physician in Indian society seems different from that of his Greek counterpart to the extent that there was some effort on the part of the brahmins to exclude medical practice and physicians from society because, as Chattopadhyaya has shown, physicians were considered by brahmins to be polluted by their association with the sick and lower classes of society. However this may be, the ayurvedic physicians continued to exist, to develop their skills and to serve their society, as *Caraka* and its companion texts and successors plainly show.

By contrast, in ancient Greece both the Hippocratic doctors and the philosophers lay outside the traditional religious conventions, but could be accepted as respected members of society, although the status of physicians was somewhat ambiguous. Some could be associated with the aristocracy, for example, Eryximachus; while others were of lower status. Some may have been famous and renowned, or at least held a fairly stable position as employed by the state, while others had to be content with a peripatetic life.

---

128. Sharma and Dash (1995), 445-447 Sūtrasthāna XXVI, verse 3-8.
129. See Lloyd "Adversaries and Authorities" (1994). Lloyd is comparing Greek and Chinese traditions, but by not taking into account early Indian medicine and science, he leaves the impression that Chinese represent 'Eastern' as opposed to 'Western' methods and that the two are fundamentally different.

The source texts of these two traditions of healing differ also in that with the Hippocratic *Corpus*, we have a collection of treatises by different authors with different purposes in mind. Some are carefully crafted polemics defending the practices of one school against another. Some are perhaps lectures or lecture notes given to student physicians. Others are the practical notebooks recording carefully observed disease processes in individual cases, or helpful reminders of what to look out for (*Epidemics, Aphorisms*). Still others are concerned with the precepts and the right conduct of the physician with his patients. Some may represent a form of practice among some physicians which was part of a wider philosophic or religious practice (*The Oath, Laws, Nutriment*).[130]

In contrast, the text of *Caraka*, although perhaps based on many separate traditions and practices, has the look of one homogenous system because it already has been compiled and redacted from these. It is the distillation of previous centuries of knowledge and accepted 'good practice'. In addition, its homogenous appearance may have something to do with a more typically Indian high regard for continuity.

Another apparent contrast is that whether for the reasons Chattopadhyaya explains or not,[131] the text incorporates explicitly both its philosophical orientation and magico-religious therapeutics, such as mantras, the uses of gems, amulets, along with more rational therapeutics and explanations of disease and health. As we have seen, some of the works in the Hippocratic *Corpus* have been viewed as generally free of recourse to the supernatural in explaining the causes or designing treatments for diseases. These have been the most valued by many scholars. This is what is usually used as proof that they are proto-scientific.[132] However, while it is true that therapeutic incantations and amulets are not found in the writings and indeed are specifically derided in some, it is not necessarily true that

130. In the Pythagorean school, however, it is very hard to separate the original sayings of Pythagoras from those of his successors because subsequent teachings are attributed to him also. Rather like Agniveśa, Pythagoras was considered by his followers to be semi-divine. See Guthrie (1967) vol. I 148-149.

131. Chattopadhyaya (1979) c. 2.

132. E.g. *Ancient Medicine, The Sacred Disease*.

awareness of 'higher' agencies at work is not to be found in the *Corpus*. There is evidence that at least some at least of Hippocratic physicians recognised the existence of divine powers which may have their part to play in the outcome of the disease. One treatise, *Regimen IV* (LXXXIX), bases its treatment on the understanding of the patient's dreams as divine in origin, or related to the movements of the stars and planets.[133] Thus in this respect the two traditions may be considered to have a similar awareness of the broader, non-material context in which individual illness occurs.

Sharma, one of the modern translators of *Caraka*, notes in his introduction that

> Āyurveda in general and *Caraka* in particular attach considerable importance to the intimate relationship between the mind (mental activities) and the body (physical functions). Any disturbance in the one affects the other and causes diseases. Therefore for the maintenance of positive health as well as for cure of diseases, both mind and the body are required to be kept in proper condition.[134]

It is doubtful that Sharma, writing in the early 1970s, could have had in mind the term 'holistic medicine' which it is used today, but his words succinctly describe the basis and aims of this approach, with its emphasis on the necessity to consider not only the body but the part that mind and emotions play in physical disease, and its equal emphasis on prevention and health maintenance. Āyurveda has had this inclination since its earliest times, perhaps because of its early association with the heterodox ascetic tradition and it has maintained this attitude throughout its history. Hippocratic medicine, too, shows an association with early Western philosophers, sharing in the view that human beings are a microcosm of a greater, divine, intelligent macrocosm. It remains to examine in more detail how this mind-body-spirit connection is evident in the earliest records of the two medical traditions.

133. Some dreams are atributed to divine origins (Jones (1979) vol. IV 423, 435) some are repetitions of daytime thoughts and actions (beneficial); some are contrary to the actions of the day and are bad in that they disturb the body; some are caused by surfeited secretion.

134. Sharma and Dash (1995) vol. I xxxiii.

CHAPTER 2

# A SURVEY OF EVIDENCE OF HOLISM IN THE HIPPOCRATIC *CORPUS* AND *CARAKA SAṂHITĀ*

Having introduced a general background of the culture of the sixth and fifth centuries B.C. with respect to medicine, we may proceed with our enquiry into the existence of any concepts in these ancient traditions which relate to those in contemporary holistic medicine. This chapter will survey the Hippocratic *Corpus* for evidence of these characteristics, and will then compare these with any corresponding ideas in *Caraka*. As with the characteristics outlined in the Introduction, although an effort is made to separate them out as a means of discussion, in reality each aspect is so much part of the others that several ideas are often found together within a single passage.

## Vital Force

The first of our characteristics is that holism takes as its premise some intelligent life principle underlying the created universe, often called the vital force, conceived as a subtle energy in the human body. In health, disease and treatment this principle is recognised by holistic practitioners, worked with, and considered ultimately responsible for energising the healing of the body. What evidence is there that this idea was present in the fifth and fourth centuries B.C. among the physicians of ancient Greece?

Reading the treatises, we may at first conclude that there is little or none. With the exception perhaps of *Breaths*, none discusses explicitly in detail any underlying philosophical concepts about how the world was created and maintained. Some seem explicitly to refute or disparage any such 'philosophical' influence in medicine. Many of the treatises are rigorously practical, concerned with strict observation and record keeping; others describe disease processes in detail, along with their treatments. Some authors argue to establish or defend the uniqueness and worthiness of medicine as a *techne* or art among the other valued arts and sciences. The arguments by the author of *The Sacred Disease* that a disease could not be caused by gods, and his dismissal of charm sellers could be taken as evidence that the Hippocratic physicians outrightly refused any recognition of a non-material aspect in disease and healing.

Yet a closer reading of the treatises shows that in many there is recognition of the fundamental holistic principle. As has been discussed in the previous chapter, there was a close relationship between these physicians and the philosophic concepts being developed at that time. Many of these concepts showed a recognition of an underlying divine principle in the world and within man.[1] In certain Hippocratic treatises there are concepts grounded in a similar acceptance of a universal divine creative principle manifested in the individual human being, sometimes as 'air', *aer* or *pneuma*, sometimes as 'soul', *psuche*, sometimes as 'nature', *phusis*. In the context of the medical writers, 'divine' suggests less the anthropomorphic deities (although occassional mention is made of 'the gods'), and demons, or magical powers. It primarily refers to that which is the eternal, creative principle, the *arche* of the universe, which was also present in the human body.[2]

A powerful example from the author of *The Sacred Disease* reflects the general philosophic outlook: phenomena are natural, divine and also rational: the text states that "all diseases are natural and all divine."[3] This establishes that a divine force is implicit in the world, a world which is both natural and orderly (or rational) and which includes the human organism. Even

1. According to Temkin (1995) 189, "the philosophers de-mythologised the gods and identified the divine with nature as a power ruling the universe with immanent necessity."
2. Lain Entralgo (1970) 148. "The *phusis* of the body is the principle *arche* of the *logos* in medicine." Compare Potter (1995) vol. VIII 21-23: "The nature of the body is the beginning point of medical reasoning."
3. Jones (1972) vol. II 183.

disease, which is ultimately inimical to life, is part of this order. For this physician as for the philosophers, the natural and divine are not separate.

Similarly, for the author of *Breaths*, there is a universal principle which he names as *aer* and *pneuma*, the source of life, health and also disease. He states,

> For what can take place without it? In what is it not present? What does it not accompany?..there is nothing that is empty of air... for mortals too this is the cause of life and the cause of disease in the sick. (III, IV).[4]

Several authors use the term *psuche*. This word is problematic when it comes to translations and interpretation, and as Onians has shown holds slightly different meanings for different writers. For example, it can be translated as 'soul', implying a spiritual, divine entity but also 'mind', implying strictly mental faculties, or possibly what we today would mean by 'psychology', a mental-emotional dimension. Onians traces a transition from the life-soul in Homer and Hesiod to its associations with perception, thought and feelings which were formerly attributed to the chest region (*thumos, phrenes* and *ker*). It is by various writers associated with breath and rooted in the marrow (Democritus), with the seed (Leucippus), with the conscious element as air (Diogenes of Apollonia).[5] Empedocles distinguised between the *psuche* as vital warmth which returns on death to the fiery element and *daimon*. *Daimon* had nothing to do with perception or thought but was an 'occult' self, capable of re-incarnation and the carrier of man's potential divinity as well as present guilt.[6] It is difficult to tell exactly which meaning is carried for each author of the treatises but for our purposes what is relevant is that its use in some texts signals that the physicians recognised a special faculty in man, a consciousness which was connected to or implicit in both the material body and the divine or spiritual dimension.

For the author of *Regimen I*, the divine and the natural are interwoven in man, each influencing the other. The soul, to the extent it is thought divine, is unchanging but, at least in the

4. Ibid., 231.
5. Onians (1994) 116-117.
6. Dodds (1951) 153.

human body, it also consists of the material substances of fire and water. "Man is of fire and water." (III) and "into man there enters a soul having fire and water" (VII). "All things are set in due order both the soul of man and likewise his body." (VI) "Soul is the same in all living creatures, although the body of each is different" (XXVIII).

> All things both human and divine are in a state of flux upwards... things of the other world do the work of this and those of this world do the work of that ... all things take place for them [men] through a divine necessity (V) "Soul is always alike...[it] changes neither through nature or force.[7]

*Regimen IV,* LXXXVI also recognises an interplay between soul and body. The soul is affected by the body, but has a separate existence and its own consciousness and sphere of activity.

> When the body is awake the soul is its servant and is never her own mistress but divides her attention among many things.... But when the body is at rest, the soul, being set in motion and awake, administers her own household and of herself performs all acts of the body. For...the soul when awake has cognisance of all things ... all functions of body and soul are performed by the soul during sleep. Whoever knows how to interpret these acts aright knows a great part of wisdom.[8]

Even the predominantly practical observations recorded by the author of *Epidemics* 6 recognise a mutual influence between the soul (divine force) and the physical disease. "The soul of man grows until death. If the soul be burnt up with a disease, it consumes the body." (6, 2)[9]

## Nature

Another term which the physicians used which implies a recognition of a fundamental creative principle or energy is

7. Jones (1979) vol. IV 231, 241, 239, 267, 237, 267.
8. Ibid., 421-423 compare also with *Regimen I,* c. II.
9. Smith (1994) vol. VII 255.

*phusis*, nature. As Temkin has pointed out 'nature', *phusis*, is in essence the divine principle: originator of life and active in maintaining life, or when imbalanced, responsible for disease.

> The divine is repeatedly mentioned in the Hippocratic writings and is often identified with what we call natural... The concept of nature and its close relationship to thought about the divine were so deeply grounded in Hippocratic medical thinking as to force the question of whether Hippocratic medicine was inseparably bound to a religion of nature.... The notion of nature as a principle of order, regularity and normalcy, open to observation and rational calculation, was fundamental for Hippocratic medicine.[10]

It is this principle of divine nature, responsible for the rational order and regularity of the physical world, that was wondered at and pondered over.[11] *Kosmos*, the Greek' word for order, is also the term used for this universal and divine order, the whole of the natural world. Nature is the healing, life-promoting power in this world. For the Greeks there would have been no question of humans not being part of nature. This was a common and deeply ingrained way of thinking and talking about the world.[12] For the physician's nature was

> the real and truly divine... before which man must prostrate himself in veneration...theirs was a physiological piety more or less harmoniously united with the cult of the traditional gods and accepted by the authors of the Hippocratic collection.[13]

Such convictions can be found in the collection in the following examples:

*Epidemics* 6.5, 1 states:

> The body's nature is the physician in disease. Nature finds the way for herself, not from thought [or: without

10. Temkin (1995) 188-190.
11. Sigerist (1961) 88.
12. Lloyd (1991) 424.
13. Lain Entralgo cited by Temkin (1995) 188 from *La medicina hipocrática* (1970) 57.

> having been taught]....Well trained, readily and without instruction, nature does what is needed.[14]

Likewise, the author of *Nutriment* believes "Nature is sufficient in all for all" (XV); that "The natures of all are untaught" (XXXIX); and that for the physician it is "necessary to deal with nature from without and within". (XVI)[15]

*Regimen I*, XV states that

> ...to do away with that which causes pain, and by taking away the cause of his suffering [*ponei*] to make him sound [literally healthy, *hugiea*]. Nature of herself knows how to do these things.[16]

These examples reveal that the physicians not only recognised the power of this divine force, but saw this principle as inherently intelligent—knowing what to do, how to do it— working for the best, even if sometimes this meant ultimately recovery was not possible: "If nature is in opposition, everything is in vain", writes the author of *Law* in chapter II.[17]

Knowledge of nature is the basis of the physician's skill and art. Some physicians may have considered it a holy, or sacred pursuit. Nature, in this context seems not confined to the physical level but includes the spiritual as well.

> Things however that are holy are revealed only to men who are holy. The profane may not learn them until they have been initiated into the mysteries of science,

concludes the author of *Law* (V).[18]

---

14. Smith (1994) vol. VII 255.
15. Jones (1972) vol. I 347, 357, 347.
16. Jones (1979) vol. IV 253.
17. Jones (1981) vol. II 263.
18. Ibid., 265. Jones has translated *epistemes* as "science" but it can also mean "knowledge, wisdom, understanding, experience, skill" and in this context it may be possible that it has the connotation of true knowledge in the sense of awareness of a higher—i.e., eternal, divine—level of being, such as for example, Plato's Forms. A suggestion of such an awareness is also found in *Regimen* I, IV: "They trust the eyes rather than the mind.... But I use mind to expound thus. For there is life in the things of the other world as well as those of this" (vol. IV 235).

## Disease is One: Disturbance in the Natural Harmony of the Body

Another of our characteristics of holistic medicine was its concept of disease. Disease may manifest itself in many different ways and places in the body and can appear to be separate, individual diseases. Many individual diseases are identified, recorded, and discussed at length in the *Corpus*: various types of fevers, dropsy, phrenitis, epilepsy, consumption, for example. However, ultimately it is in fact one in its origins. The author of *Breaths* exemplifies the physicians' approach: while there are individual diseases, underlying these is one basic cause of all, disturbance of the harmonious flow of the vital force. Chapter II states, "Now of all diseases the fashion is the same, but the seat varies. So while diseases are thought to be entirely unlike one another, owing to the difference in their seat, in reality all have one essence, and cause." In the next two passages he reveals this essence as *aer*. "It is the most powerful of all and in all...." It is said to be a 'current' and a 'flowing', invisible but present and the cause of life and of disease.[19]

For the author of *Nature of Man* disease is disturbance of the fundamental harmony or proper mixture among the different humours or elements of the organism. In *Ancient Medicine* it is improper mixing of factors, particularly of tastes, which upsets the body's harmony; the acrid, sweet, salty are said to make up the human organism. For the author of *Regimen I* it is a disturbance to the balance among food, digestion and exercise, between repletion and depletion, between consumption and evacuation via urine, sweat or stool. For each author any disturbance in the basic, natural balance of fundamental factors is the cause of disease. Even more, it is this imbalance, the real disease, which must be treated, not only results of the imbalance, i.e., the manifestations of individual diseases and symptoms.

## The Wisdom of the Body: The Self-healing Mechanism

As the above references show, disease and health are dynamic processes, opposite sides of the same coin. The vital force, as

19. Ibid., 229, 231 *cheuma* and *rheuma*.

nature or as *pneuma* is capable of being the cause of disease when the body becomes unbalanced, or its flow is blocked. But this force is also the healer of the body, when its benevolent balance is restored. This healing propensity is entirely within the normal function of the human organism. Nature acts "without having been taught." This self-healing effort, which is seen as automatic, is observed by the physicians as the body's *ponos.*[20] This word means both suffering or pain, and toil or work. Thus the symptoms of disease, such as bleeding, loose stools, abscesses, fevers are understood not only as the body's suffering but also as the body's working to restore balance. In terms of the Hippocratics, the body's various excretions and secretions were the chief means of this self-help. They observed the body naturally doing these things as part of its work, *ponos* against disease, since it was such things as these which restored the balance. Heat is also seen as acting to concoct or ripen and remix the raw and separated humours so that the body's natural state of balance is restored. Fever itself was sometimes seen as an example of the body's healing effort.[21] Sometimes one ailment supervening on another helps cure it. For example, in *Aphorisms* VI, XI and XXI the appearance of haemorrhoids effects the cure of mania, melancholy and kidney infections. Such cleansing activities are understood as nature's ways of ridding the body of its impurities [22] through a release mechanism. This is an important aspect of the work of self-healing.

---

20. This concept is not declared explicitly by the writers, but is suggested by many passages. It was highlighted by Seyle (1984) 11, and it can be found in such passages as *Ancient Medicine* XVI-XVIII where the author argues that the body spontaneously produces cold to counteract heat and vice versa, and that flows (eliminations) of humours are beneficial if they are concocted. *Epidemics* I, XV notes the beneficial effects of spontaneous stools, and haemorrhage on fevers. *Humours* XX states, "All other abscessions, too, such as fistula, are cures of other diseases. So symptoms that relieve complaints if they come after their development, prevent the development if they come before" Jones (1979) 93. Thus the manifestation of symptoms reflects the body's effort at elimination of the cause of the disease, whether preventatively or after the establishment of the disease.
21. Neuburger (1932) 7 Neuburger cites the following: *Aphorism* IV, LVII; *Aphorisms* VI, XL; *Aphorisms* VII, LII (e.g., "When there is severe pain in the liver, if fever supervenes it removes the pain"); *Aphorisms* V, LXX: a quartan fever cures convulsions; *Epidemics* VI, VI.5 (quartan fever can cure epilepsy).
22. Jones (1979) footnote 2, vol. IV 183.

Such releasing efforts are referred to as purging or cleansing, words which may have some religious connotations. However such connotations seem not to be present for the physicians in the religious sense that the disease is seen as a sin for which the sufferer has to be punished.

## The Mind–Body Connection

Today with our increased knowledge about how mental and emotional processes affect the most minute body functions via the hormonal and nervous systems, we have secured concrete, material proof that a person's mental and emotional state can predispose toward disease, even trigger it. Some of the passages already cited have suggested that the Hippocratic physician, though lacking much detail of anatomy and physiology, was nonetheless well aware of this relationship. Others are more explicit and show how they incorporated it into their therapy.

Although such passages are relatively few compared to those which deal with the more practical aspects of the profession, none the less such an awareness is evident and shows that some writers were fully cognisant of the mind-body-spirit whole. The fact that these passages were thought important enough to be preserved argues that they were important to ancient physicians.

One example is from the author of *Epidemics* 6.5,5. He notes that

> Anger contracts the heart and the lungs and draws the hot and the moist substances into the head. Contentment releases the heart *and those substances* [emphasis mine].

The mental-emotional state directly affects the physical, initiating release of the excess heat and moist material. He demonstrates an understanding of the multiplicity of factors necessary to health, including the mental ones when he goes on to state, "Labour is food for the joints and the flesh, sleep for the intestines. Intellection is a stroll for the soul in men."[23]

The concept of man being constituted of a blending and mixing of humours or elements was not necessarily confined to the

23. Smith (1994) vol. VII 257.

physical level, as the following passages from *Regimen I*, show. Again 'soul' here may suggest both mind/consciousness and spirit. That the physical interacts with the mental-spiritual is suggested by the remedy given for a mind that rushes about too much: the remedy is dietary.

> XXXV: 'But it is not beneficial for such to use wrestling, massage or like exercises, for fear lest the pores becoming hollow, they be filled with surfeit. For the motion of the soul is of necessity weighed down by such things.... For the senses of the soul that act through sight or hearing are quick; while those that act through touch are slower, and produce a deeper impression....If the fire have a pure blend, the body is healthy and such a soul is intelligent... For if his body be in a healthy state and be not troubled from any source, the blend of his soul is intelligent....But if the power of water be further mastered by the fire, the soul must be quicker... and on account of its speed rushes on to too many objects. Such a person is benefited by a regimen inclining more to water than the preceding; he must eat barley bread rather than wheaten and fish rather than meat.'[24]

XXXVI continues, "It is this blending, then, that is, as I have now explained, the cause of the soul's intelligence or want of it; regimen can make this blending either better or worse."[25]

The author of *Breaths*, held that intelligence, consciousness and the air principle embodied as breath were intimately connected to body substances. In Chapter XIV, he observes that "when the blood alters, the intelligence also changes".[26]

*Epidemics* 6.8,10 says that "even the mind's consciousness, itself by itself, distant from the organs and events feels misery, joy, is fearful and optimistic, feels hope and despair. Like the servant of Hippothous, although by herself in her mind she was conscious of the things that followed on her disease."[27]

---

24. Jones (1979) vol. IV 285, 287, 289.
25. Ibid., 293.
26. Jones (1981) vol. II 249 for intelligence, *phronesis*.
27. Smith (1994) vol. VII 281, 283 for consiousness, *gnomes xunnoia;* for mind, *gnomes*.

This passage, especially the last statement, Phillips points out, shows that a person could divine the progress of her illness through an 'internal sense', an intuitive knowledge of the body, not aided by external observation or by the physician, and this sense, the mind's consciousness, "was something of itself which determined all the feelings."[28]

The author of *Humours* recognised 'psychic symptoms' indicated by the patient's behaviour.

> Among psychical symptoms are intemperance in drink and food, in sleep and in wakefulness, the endurance of toil either for the sake of certain passions ... or of one's craft or of necessity, and the regularity or irregularity of such endurance.

Thus when a person's lifestyle or behaviour change from what is normal and natural, such signs, though not manifesting as a full blown disease state, were important as indicators of a preliminary stage to disease for they reveal a disturbance of the internal harmony of the psyche.[29] The remedy accordingly can be to change from negative patterns to positive ones. *Aphorisms* II, XLV notes that "Epilepsy among the young is cured chiefly by change—change of age, of climate, of place, of mode of life."[30]

*Humours* goes on to be quite clear that mental states and emotions are directly affected by change and are responded to by changes in the physical organs.

> States of mind before and after changes.... Fears, shame, pain, pleasure, passion ... to each of these the appropriate member of the body responds by its action. Instances are sweats, the palpitation of the heart and so forth.

He also notes that disharmony or disease can originate in either body or consciousness: "For coughs, like fevers, cause abcessions. These results are the same whether they come from humours, or from wasting of body and soul" (IX).[31]

---

28. Phillips (1973) 72.
29. Jones (1979) vol. IV 81.
30. Ibid., 119 mode of life, *bion*.
31. Ibid., 81.

*Aphorisms* VI, XXVII attributes melancholia to prolonged fear and depression.

The author of *The Sacred Disease*, gives perhaps the most eloquent account of the concept that all disease ultimately is of one cause, disturbance in all powerful *aer–pneuma*, and that it affects the whole body, starting first with the mind or brain, the seat of intelligence and consciousness, because it is the first to receive the all powerful *aer*.

> In these ways I hold that the brain is the most powerful organ of the human body, for when it is healthy it is an interpreter to us of the phenomena caused by the air, as it is the air that gives it intelligence. Eyes, ear, tongue, hands and feet act in accordance with the discernment of the brain; in fact the whole body participates in intelligence in proportion to its participation in air. To consciousness the brain is the messenger. For when a man draws breath into himself, the air first reaches the brain and so is dispersed through the rest of the body, though it leaves in the brain its quintessence... (XIX).[32]
>
> Men ought to know that from the brain and from the brain only, arise our pleasures, joys, laughter and jests, as well as our sorrows, pains, griefs and tears...it is the same thing which makes us mad or delirious, inspires us with dread and fear, whether by night or by day, brings sleeplessness, inopportune mistakes, aimless anxieties, absent-mindedness and acts which are contrary to habit. These things that we suffer all come from the brain, when it is not healthy but becomes abnormally hot, cold, moist or dry or suffers any other unnatural affection to which it was not accustomed...all the time the brain is still a man is intelligent (XVII).[33]

*The Sacred Disease* recognises that the heart and diaphragm also reflect the emotions, but the brain, as seat of consciousness, is of ultimate importance:

---

32. Ibid., vol. II 179.
33. Ibid., 175.

> The body must, too, when in pain, shiver and be strained and the same effects are produced by excess of joy, because the heart and the diaphragm are best endowed with feeling.

But the brain is the more important in terms of its effects on the entire body, for the author continues

> neither, however, has any share of intelligence [higher awareness] but it is the brain which is the cause of all the things I have mentioned...it is the first of the bodily organs to perceive the intelligence coming from the air, so too if any violent change has occurred in the air owing to the seasons, the brain also becomes different from what it was. Therefore I assert that the diseases too that attack it are the most acute, most serious, most fatal, and the hardest for the inexperienced to judge of (XX).[34]

The last aphorism of the *Corpus* also most eloquently expresses the understanding of an intelligent consciousness or soul permeating the body until the time of death.

> The boundary of death is passed when the heat of the soul has risen above the navel to the part above the diaphragm, and all the moisture has been burnt up...there passes away all at once the breath of the heat (wherefrom the whole was constructed) into the whole again, partly through the flesh and partly through the breathing organs in the head, whence we call it the 'breath of life'. And the soul leaving the tabernacle of the body, gives up the cold, mortal image to bile, blood, phlegm and flesh.[35]

## Treating the Body via the Mind

Treatments most often mentioned even for mental disturbances, whether from fevers or from fears and depressions were by material means, usually cleansing with herbs, taken internally or applied externally, or by massage or diet. However, there is some evidence that the physicians also realised that the physical body could also be affected by addressing the mind and emotions and

34. Ibid., 181. Note the observation of how even seasonal changes affect consciousness.
35. Jones, 1979 vol. IV 219, 221.

occasionally had recourse to such treatment. The physician of *Regimen IV*, a treatise which takes into account the influence of the motions of the heavenly bodies and of dreams on the patient, actually recommends as treatment that a patient attend comic theatrical performances, perhaps the first instance of 'laughter therapy' recently made famous and credible by Norman Cousins.[36] The physician advises in chapter LXXXIX:

> Rest is beneficial in such a case. The soul should be turned to the contemplation of comic things, if possible, if not to such other things as will bring most pleasure when looked at, for two or three days, and recovery will take place.[37]

**Healing involves participation on the part of the patient and the physician. The patient takes responsibility and engages in the healing process. The physician treats the individual in his or her wholeness not just the specific diseased body part**

The patient is responsible for his or her own healing process since the human organism, far from being over and above nature, is recognised by the Hippocratic physicians as intimately interrelated to its inner and outer environment. This is the very basis for their use of dietetics, herbs, advice on exercise and lifestyle habits, and their *prognostikon* and understanding of the patient's individual *phusis* or constitution, his individual blend of the fundamental factors.

This precept is a corollary to observing the self-healing of the body. The patient can help or hinder this automatic healing force by such things as lifestyle, diet, exercises/rest and mental attitude, and by following the advice of the physician.

We read for example in *Aphorisms* I, I that "the physician must be ready not only to do his duty but to secure the co-operation of the patient, the attendant and of externals."[38] *Regimen in Acute Diseases* LXVI advises "Let the habits of the patient carry great

36. Cousins (1981). Cousin's experience has been followed up. According to Patch Adams ("Laughter Medicine", Feather stone and Forsyth (1997), 315-321) scientists are studying the effects of laughter on the body; several hospitals are bringing humour into the medical programme, and an Association of Therapeutic Humours exists.
37. Jones (1979) vol. IV 433.
38. Ibid., 99.

weight."[39] *Nature of Man* recognises that "The patient himself must bring about a cure by combating the cause of the disease, for in this way will be removed that which caused the disease in the body" (XIII).[40] The author of *The Art* points out that patients bear ultimate responsibility for their condition and their recovery:

> What escapes the eyesight is mastered by the eye of the mind, and the sufferings of the patients, due to their not being quickly observed are the fault, not of the medical attendants, but of the nature of the patient and of the disease...if they understood their diseases, they would never have fallen into them (XI).[41]

This passage reflects on both the patient and the physician. It recalls the viewpoint of Socrates that if men could or would know the Good, they would automatically act in a just and good way. If the patient were more knowledgeable about his/her body and how it was feeling, he might be able to keep it from reaching a diseased state. It also reveals that the physicians felt that their training in *logikon* and practical experience had enabled them to see beneath the superficial state of affairs with the 'eye of the mind' to the true reality of the patient's condition.[42] Physicians felt this ability distinguished their understanding from that of the layman. The quote from *Regimen* I, IV cited above also shows this attitude, and hints even that with the right mental training, another level of reality beyond that knowable by the physical senses can be attained.[43]

If, or once the patient becomes aware of his condition he can do a lot to help him or herself. *Humours* V points out that "helpful

---

39. Jones (1981) vol. II 123.
40. Jones (1979) vol. IV 37.
41. Jones (1981) vol. II 211.
42. Jones (1981) vol. II 209. "Without doubt no man who sees only with his eyes can know anything of what has been here described [the internal organs and structures]...Their obscurity, however, does not mean they are our masters...for what escapes the eyesight is mastered by the eye of the mind (*gnomes opsei*).
43. Perhaps such attitudes were among those that invited Plato to use the medical reasoning as a model for, or example of what he was trying to communicate as regards the soul. For an example of another see Smith (1979) 48, 49. Referring to the *Phaedrus*, 269d, Smith writes, "Plato sees a parallel between Hippocrates' *gnosis* and *diagnosis* (which mean "know together" and "know separately") and his own collection and division".

abscessions must be encouraged by food, drinks, smells, sights, sounds, ideas, evacuations, warmth, cooling ...plaster, salves, sleep."[44]

*Ancient Medicine* notes it is very important to engage the patient in the healing process, and has every faith in his ability to respond:

> It is particularly necessary for one who discusses this art to discuss things familiar to ordinary folk. For the subject of inquiry and discussion is simply and solely the sufferings of these same ordinary folk. Now to learn by themselves how their own sufferings come about and cease, and the reasons why they get worse or better is not an easy task for ordinary folk, but when these things have been discovered and are set forth by another, it is simple...But if you miss being understood by laymen, and fail to put your hearers in this condition, you will miss reality (II).[45]

## Treatment of the Individual

The concept of the individual constitution or *phusis* we find in the treatises most reveals the conviction among physicians that each patient must be treated individually, taking into account the many aspects of life, both internal and external, the mental-emotional as well as the physical, that are constantly influencing the organism. This subject will be discussed in more detail in chapter four. The Hippocratic physicians showed a remarkable sensitivity to the effects of stress, i.e., any change or upset from what is normal and natural on the human organism, and fully realised that this is the cause of the essential disturbance of the body's natural harmony, the fundamental cause of disease. Being convinced that man's health mirrored, and was enhanced by following the order and regularity of the cycles of nature, whether great or small, they usually spoke of this in terms of anything which caused a disturbance in *diaita* or *bios*, the mode of living – the habits and natural rhythms of life, whether these be in emotions, state of mind, seasons, climate, foods, labour, rest or exercise.

---

44. Jones (1979) vol. IV 73.
45. Jones (1972) vol. I 15, 17 for reality, *ontas*.

Sometimes the slightest alteration in such habits could set the stage for disease. "Instability is characteristic of the humours, and so they may be easily altered by nature and by chance" (*Decorum* XIII).[46]

*Ancient Medicine* dwells particularly on the changes in food intake as causes for disease. For the author of *Nature of Man* the cause is anything which alters the balance of humours.

Also, unusual or traumatic events or experiences were understood to cause the disturbance which leads to disease. "It is changes that are chiefly responsible for diseases, especially the greatest changes, the violent alterations both in seasons and in other things" (*Humours* XV).[47]

> So in all cases all the evidence concurs in proving that all sudden changes, that depart widely from the mean in either direction, are injurious (*Regimen in Acute Diseases*, XLVI).[48]

*The Sacred Disease* states that we suffer diseases when the brain "suffers any other unnatural affection to which it was not accustomed" (XVII).[49] Even a shock or fright is understood to disturb the entire body by 'chilling' it. Epilepsy in children can be caused by a chilling wind or

> by fear of the mysterious, if the patient be afraid at a shout, or if while weeping he be unable quickly to recover his breath.... Whichever of them occur he is immediately chilled, the patient loses the power of speech and does not breathe, the breath stops, the brain hardens, the blood stays, and so the phlegm separates off and flows down (XIII).[50]

*Regimen in Acute Diseases*, VI warns the physician to pay great attention to the details of the patient's lifestyle: "Let the habits of the patient carry great weight".[51]

---

46. Jones (1981) vol. II 295.
47. Jones (1979) vol. IV 89.
48. Jones (1981) vol. II 103.
49. Ibid., 175.
50. Ibid., 167.
51. Ibid., 123.

## The Physician's Role

Within this view of the healing power of nature and the patient's participation, the physician's role is to work with, to support or encourage what the body is trying to do anyway. This does not mean, however, that the physicians saw their task as merely to sit by, observe and record; nor did they find that the means of help at their disposal were ineffective. On the contrary, their experience gave them confidence that with training, and a particular method of reasoning they could discern the cause of the imbalance. Using a variety of therapeutic strategies which mimicked what nature was doing, they could restore balance. The Hippocratic physician would have understood that blocking this self-healing mechanism (for example, the fever or inflammation) while welcome as relieving suffering temporarily, would be interfering with this mechanism and would not address the underlying cause of the disease nor bring about the re-establishment of the body's harmony and health. This would be treating merely the part and not the 'whole body'.

The physician is seen as acting in concert with nature's healing force to restore wholeness, the shared goal. One author compares his role to other creative craftsmen such as cobblers:

> Cobblers divide wholes into parts and make the parts wholes; cutting and stitching they make sound what is rotten. Man too has the same experience. Wholes are divided into parts, and from union of the parts wholes are formed. By stitching and cutting, that which is rotten in men is healed by the physician's art: to do away with that which causes pain, and by taking away the cause of his suffering to make him sound. Nature of herself knows how to do these things.... In other respects too nature is the same as the physician's art" (*Regimen I*, XV).[52]

For some Hippocratic physicians this engagement with the divine principles of nature was a discipline of living and working in accordance with the natural order of the universe.

---

52. Ibid., vol. IV 253 wholes, *hola*; sound, healthy, *hugeia*.

The author of *Decorum* (V) writes "For the physician who is a lover of wisdom is the equal of a god."[53]

Viewed from the vantage point of the twenty-first century with its highly developed medicines and medical technology the therapeutic methods employed by Hippocratic physicians may seem at first ineffective, but at least harmless: the resort of those who had little else to offer. However, seen within the context of their model of medicine, the treatment followed a carefully worked out rationale and, as far as the evidence of the physicians' experience proved, worked well, although not successfully all the time. In addition, on the evidence of similar practices found in ancient Ayurvedic medicine and still in use today, the Hippocratic therapeutics may be reassessed as being similarly effective, and worth being judiciously applied in the modern world.[54]

Part of the physicians' skill and training involved learning to discern which patients were capable of responding to treatment. This art of *prognostikon* not only guided the physician in judging whether to take on the patient but helped him understand the likely course of the disease and suggested the best treatment method. "Furthermore, he will carry out the treatment best if he know beforehand from the present symptoms what will take place later" (*Prognostic*, I). Of course, such a skill was open to abuse and physicians were not always thought of highly, but for the writers of the *Corpus*, *prognostikon* was a valuable part of their art, intended for the good of the patient as well as the physician. It was part of helping the patient according to his individual *phusis*.

> It is necessary to learn the natures of such diseases, how they exceed the strength of men's bodies and to learn how to forecast them (*Prognostic*, I).[55]

It was also used to gain the confidence of the patient.

The physician, the passage from *Prognostic* suggests, was alert to many signs which gave him clues about the patient's entire

53. Ibid., vol. II 287.
54. In fact, they are, among many herbalists and naturopaths. Bastyr University in Seattle has an accredited syllabus to train naturopathic physicians.
55. Ibid., 7-9.

lifestyle and history, so that he did not have to rely exclusively on what the patient told him. He seems to have been rather like Sherlock Holmes, noticing everything and using it to piece out the history and circumstances of the case. For example, the author discusses how the face looks, whether the patient shuns the light, how he is found to be lying, whether grinding the teeth is a habit from childhood or something new. Such things are mentioned in addition to the acute observations about the disease itself, its symptoms, the signs of urine, sputum, the periods and crises of the fevers. The age of the patient, and nature of the weather and seasons is also important to know, as these are known to affect the cause, nature and progress of the disease.

## Treatments for the Whole Body

We have noted the physician sometimes prescribed experiences which would influence the mind and therefore the body of the patient. Among the more physical treatments recommended in the *Corpus* were diet, exercise, massage, drugs, fomentations, vapour baths, baths, blood letting, cautery and surgery. Except perhaps for these last two, their applications were an attempt to follow what nature was striving for anyway: cleansing the body by means of "excretions and secretions" and/or heating or ripening the humours and "leading" them out of the body. For example, cleansing was done by means of sweating with diaphoretic herbs taken internally to promote sweating in the body generally, or by means of fomentations of aromatic herbs over locally affected parts. The stomach was cleansed by emetics. Cleansing the bowels was primarily by herbs which acted as purgatives. Hellebore is often mentioned as useful for purging. That the physicians used this herb so frequently suggests they knew exactly what they were doing. Even blood letting was used following the observation that when the body spontaneously bled, it often improved the condition. It was not a therapy that was undertaken lightly nor applied without first weighing the pros and cons. Hippocratic treatments were not applied indiscriminately nor in vain hopes, but rather judiciously, i.e., used in some cases and not in others, at the right moment of the course of the disease, when the patient was strong enough; in other words, as the physician judged best. For the writers of the *Corpus*, their training, their craft of medicine prepared them with the experience and judgement to know when a treatment should be used and when not.[56]

In addition to such cleansing therapy, patients were also given special therapeutic diets (the subject of Chapter Three), prescribed either special exercises or rest, and advised as to beneficial changes in their life habits. Massage was also prescribed. The purpose of these was specifically to help restore balance, or, preventatively, to maintain the patient's inherent balance, or health.

Some examples of the above therapies and the knowledge of the physicians in their use are found in the treatises as the following examples show:

From *Epidemics 2. 3,2:*

> We know the characteristics of drugs, from what one comes what kinds of things. For they are not equally good but different characteristics are good in different circumstances. In different places medical drugs are gathered earlier or later; also the preparations differ such as drying, crushing, boiling and so on (I pass over most things [!]) and how much for each person and in what diseases, in relation to age, appearance, regimen, what kind of season, what season and how it is developing and the like.[57]

From *Epidemics III:*

> Case XV: The bowels under a stimulus, passed disordered matters;

---

56. Some of these herbs were very powerful. Hellebore, *Veratrum album*, for example, is most often mentioned for cleansing "downwards" the "lower cavity". *Aphorisms* IV, XVI cautions that hellebore produces convulsions in the healthy and is dangerous for them. Today hellebore is not used by herbalists; it is a violent irritant poison affecting the central nervous system and causing life-threatening narcotic symptoms. However, even poisons can be medicines and the difference lies in the skill with which they are used: special methods of preparation and knowing the therapeutic dose. Gold, for example, is a poison but, properly prepared and in the right dose is used today in the treatment of rheumatoid arthritis.

57. Smith (1994) vol. III 51.

Case X: Hot sweating all over; the fever passed away in a crisis;
Case XIV: Urine concocts and sweating... a perfect crisis.[58]

From *Epidemics* 6.5, 4:

Healing is a dispute with a disease, not agreement. Cold both helps and kills. The same for the effects of heat.[59]

*Affections*, 2:
If pains befall the head...warm his head by washing it with copious hot water, and to carry off phlegm and mucus by having him sneeze. If...he is not relieved, clean his head of phlegm, and prescribe a regimen of gruel and drinking water...These pains attack as the result of phlegm, when having been set in motion, it collects in the head.

*Affections*, 4:
If pain befalls the ears, ...wash with copious hot water, and administer a vapour bath to the ears.[60] ...[If this fails] have the patient drink a medication that draws phlegm upwards or to clean his head of phlegm. This pain too, is due to phlegm, when from the head it invades the ear internally.

*Affections*, 10:
It is of benefit in this disease [phrenitis, or brain fever] to wash with copious hot water from the head downwards, for as the body is softened, sweating increases, the cavity discharges, urine passes and the patient gains more control over himself.

From *Affections*, 11: In an ardent fever, from bile,
on the outside he becomes cold, but inside he is hot...administer cooling agents both to the cavity and externally...taking care he does not suffer a chill. Give drinks and gruel often, a little at a time, as cold as possible.

---

58. Jones (1972) vol. I 283, 275, 227.
59. Smith (1994) vol. VII 257 This shows the physicians applied heat and cold judiciously.
60. A vapour bath involved aiming steam to the area, probably with aromatic herbs, many of which, it is now known, have effective anti-microbial and mucolytic actions.

> Give a medication for the cavity [purge the bowels] ...also cool with very cold enemas everyday or every other day. Ardent fever arises from bile, when, having been set in motion, it is deposited inside the body; it too is liable to change into pneumonia.[61]

From *Nature of Man,* VI:

> ...a drug that withdraws bile...for when the drug enters the body, it first withdraws the constituent of the body which is most akin to itself and then it draws and purges the other constituent.[62]

*Nature of Man,* IX:

> To know the whole matter the physician must set himself against the established character of the disease, of constitutions, of seasons, and of ages.... When diseases of all sorts occur at one and the same time, it is clear that in each case the particular regimen is the cause and that the treatment carried out should be that opposed to the cause of the disease...and should be change of regimen (lifestyle, diet, exercise). This one should learn and change and carry out treatment only after examination of the patient's constitution, age, physique, the season of the year and the fashion of the disease, sometimes taking away and sometimes adding,...and so making changes in drugging or in regimen to suit the several conditions of age, season, physique and disease....[If disease is due to air, i.e., an epidemic] they should not change their regimen... but regimen should be used in this way when it manifestly does no harm to a patient...care should be taken that inspiration be of the lightest ...the place should be moved as far as possible from that in which the disease is epidemic... and the body should be reduced.[63]

Not all physicians, of course were equal in these skills, as this complaint from the author of *Regimen in Acute Diseases,* XLIII

61. Potter (1988) vol. V 11, 19-21, 21.
62. Jones (1979) vol. IV 17.
63. Ibid., 25-29.

shows:

> Nor indeed do I see that physicians are experienced in the proper way to distinguish the kinds of weakness that occur in diseases, whether it be caused by starving or by some other irritation, or by pain, or by the acuteness of the disease; the affections again, with their manifold forms, that our individual constitution and habit engender and that though a knowledge of such things brings safety and ignorance brings death.[64]

The author of *Affections* similarly reflects:

> Generally speaking it is the acute diseases that cause the most deaths and that are the most painful, and with these the greatest care and the strictest treatment are necessary. Let nothing bad be added by the person treating—rather let the evils resulting from the diseases themselves suffice—but only whatever good he is capable of. If when the physician treats correctly, the patient is overcome by the magnitude of his disease, this is not the physician's fault. But if, when the physician treats either incorrectly or out of ignorance, the patient is overcome, it is his fault.[65]

From the above passages it is clear that the ancient physicians, or at least the best of them, had quite a comprehensive understanding of the nature of disease and health and of the intricate relationship between all the factors involved and that they pursued their profession according to this understanding.

## THE HOLISTIC APPROACH OF ĀYURVEDA

Āyurveda is today considered by many people as a holistic system of healing. Rather than taking this at face value, however, it is worth exploring how its holism is expressed in the earliest treatise, the *Caraka Saṃhitā*.

Two aspects of the system which indicate a holistic approach—diet and the concept of doṣas—will be discussed in detail in the

64. Ibid., vol. II 99.
65. Potter (1988) vol. V 23-24.

following chapters. Before turning to these, we will consider some of Caraka's concepts which accord with the characteristics of holistic medicine outlined previously.

## Vital force, Mind-Body-Spirit Unity, Origins of Health and Disease

Do we find in *Caraka* a sense of a fundamental principle, a creative force, which is reflected in the myriad forms of the natural, phenomenal world; which serves as their substratum or as the link between them; which is reflected in the spirit or soul in the human organism; and whose disequilibrium is the origin of disease?

One of the eight divisions of *Caraka* is the Śārīrasthāna, a section dealing with the principles governing the creation of the universe, the human body and its physique (its composition as *dhātus* and *doṣas*), embryological development and childbirth, and the description of organs and parts of the human body. The section starts with a chapter on the 'Empirical Soul' or *puruṣa*.

In Śārīrasthāna chapter I, verses 16 and 17 *puruṣa* is defined in two different ways, the first according to the Vaiśeṣika philosophical system and the second according to a possibly old form of the Sāṃkhya philosophical system. In the first, *puruṣa* is said to comprise six elements, viz. the five *mahābhūtas* plus consciousness. In the second, *puruṣa* comprises twenty-four components: mind [*manas*], ten *indriyas* (sensory and motor organs), five objects of sense-organs and *prakṛti* or created nature, which itself consists of the five *mahābhūtas*, plus *ahaṃkāra* or individual identity or ego, intellect [*mahat*] and *avyakta*, the primordial element.[66]

Without needing to define here exactly what is meant by such terms in the different philosophical schools, we can at least see that the concepts of a soul and of a mind and its processes as manifested in, and a part of, the rational order of nature were accepted by the ancient *vaidyas*.

In verse 49 of Śārīrasthāna, the soul is distinguished from the body in the sense that "while bodily organs... might be different soul is one and the same."[67] This also suggests its link with a

66. Sharma and Dash (1994) vol. II 314.
67. Ibid., 324.

cosmic soul. Though in verses 53 and 59 the "empirical soul" or *puruṣa* is distinguished from the Absolute Soul/*paramātman* by the fact that it has a beginning and is ephemeral, it also seems more to be the case that *puruṣa* represents the aspect of the eternal that is manifested in individual human form. For the purposes of form, they are distinguished, but in essence they are the same. It is mind that is fundamentally distinguished from soul. In verses 74-76 mind is said to be active but yet devoid of consciousness, a characteristic of the soul alone.

In addition to these passages dwelling on the divine and spiritual matrix of the physical world there are others that consider how the mind and emotions play their part in disrupting the body's natural equilibrium and creating disease, i.e., Śārīrasthāna chapter II, 39-41. Verse 41 states,

> The body and mind are the seats of disease. When there is a break in the continuity of the body and mind, [i.e. when liberation of the soul is complete] then diseases cease to recur.[68]

In the first part of *Caraka*, Sūtrasthāna chapter I ("The Quest for Longevity, *Dīrghajīvitīya*"), verses 55-57 the text similarly observes that

> the body and mind constitute the substrata of diseases/*vyādhi* and happiness or positive health/*sukha* [literally, what is agreeable, comfortable]. The soul/*ātman* is essentially devoid of all pathogenicity. He is the cause of consciousness through the mind and the specific qualities of basic elements. He is eternal. He is an observer, he observes all activities. Pathogenic factors of the body are *vāyu*, *pitta* and *kapha* while those in the mind are *rajas* and *tamas*.[69]

The next verse in this chapter points out that bodily pathogenic factors are "reconciled" by religious rites and physical means (particularly diet and *drauyas*/drugs, but also massage, exercise,

68. Ibid., 362-363.
69. Ibid., vol. I 40-41. *Rajas* and *tamas* are two of the three basic qualities/*guṇas* of the mind, the active and the inert and are contrasted with a third, *sattva*, which is characterised by clarity, tranquility and harmony, a state conducive to health.

etc.) according to the principle of opposites while pathogenic factors of the mind are reconciled by spiritual and scriptural knowledge, patience, memory and meditation. The remainder of the chapter, verses 63-134, concentrates on drug therapy and discusses tastes, types of drugs (animal, vegetable, metal and minerals), and varieties of drugs in each of these categories. A drug not known (understood properly) is likened to poison, while a known drug is likened to nectar (verses 124-125). While acknowledging that religious rites have a role to play in healing, the fact that the largest part of the chapter is devoted to detailing the use of drugs suggests that this therapeutic approach is the overwhelming concern of the physician. However, the fact that such rites and spiritual knowledge and meditation are included establishes that the physicians included these in their view of what contributes to health and well-being. An example of such a holistic understanding is found in another section of *Caraka*, one dealing specifically with treatments, Cikitsāsthāna, Chapter III, verses 4 and 12. Here it states that fever, *jvara,* is the foremost among disease. "It afflicts the body, the senses and the mind"....It is caused by the three physical *doṣas* and the two mental *doṣas*, *rajas* and *tamas*."[70]

Another verse in Sūtrasthāna, chapter XI, verse 54 also considers this point: "Therapies are of three kinds; spiritual therapy, therapy based on reasoning/*yukti* (physical approach) and psychic therapy."[71] Spiritual therapy involves such practices as giving gifts or offerings, wearing amulets, the use of incantations and other ritual observances. Physical therapy involves diet and drugs. Psychic therapy involves "withdrawal of the mind from harmful objects". An example of this latter could be meditation but also perhaps, the prescription of the Hippocratic doctor for his patient to attend comic plays. Each in its way involves substituting positive thoughts and images for harmful ones. Examples of such therapies are found in Cikitsāsthāna, chapter III, verses 317-324.

Śārīrasthāna opens with the physician Agniveśa requesting Punarvasu to explain the answers to thirty questions about the

70. Ibid., vol. III 108-109.
71. Ibid., vol. I 231 and vol. III 215-216.

"Empirical Soul", its origins, whether it is eternal or ephemeral, how it becomes involved in the creation and how it is liberated from that attachment. Chapter V of Śārīrasthāna opens with a discussion on the relationship between the individual and the universe stating:

> an individual is an epitome of the universe as all the material and spiritual phenomena of the universe are present in the individual and all those present in the individual are also contained in the universe[72] (Śārīrasthāna V verses 3-4).

Of the material phenomena, the great elements (earth [*pṛthvī*], water [*jala*] fire or brilliance [*tejas*], wind or air [*vāyu*], and space [*ākāśa*]) appear in the individual in physical form as moisture, warmth, vital air or *prāṇa* and the cavities respectively. Of the spiritual phenomena, Brahman, the Absolute, is also the inner soul or *antarātman*. Thus the five great elements or *pañca-mahābbhūtas* from which the material world is derived are present in the human organism, indeed they are derived from the mind itself (Śārīrasthāna I, verse 66-67). There is a clear macrocosm–microcosm relationship.

It is most interesting that the next passage of Śārīrasthāna chapter V, paragraphs 6-7 goes on to discuss what spiritual knowledge has to do with medicine.

> One who sees equally the entire universe in his own self, and his own self in the entire universe is in possession of true knowledge/*satyā buddhi* [knowledge of one's spiritual self or Self]. Such a person experiencing the entire universe in his own self believes than none but his own self is responsible for happiness and miseries.[73]

According to the text in Śārīrasthāna V, verses 11-12, and 23-24 concerning the soul's liberation from bondage, only cessation of the soul's attachment to the physical and mental phenomena brings about "salvation" or absolute tranquillity, *praśama* or spiritual knowledge. Cessation of attachments is said to come when a person visualises the presence of everything in all

72. Ibid., vol. II 414-415.
73. Ibid., vol. II 416.

situations and is one with Brahman, the Absolute, (verse 20-21) and when the soul gets "real knowledge", i.e., realises that his identity is not with the world but with the Absolute (Śārīrasthāna I, verses 152-153).

We may pause here to note that in verses 3-5 *vāyu* is recorded as one of the five great elements and the text also states that universal *vāyu* is *prāṇa*, or breath, in the individual. Elsewhere in *Caraka*, great prominence is given to *vāyu* as the fundamental principle in the universe. In passage 8 of Sūtrasthāna XII, where the subject matter is the functions and disorders of Wind, *vāyu* is equated with the old Vedic god of wind and identified as the origin and ending of all:

> The god *Vāyu* is the eternal cause of the universe. He brings existence as well as destruction to all living beings. He causes happiness and misery...He has permeated the whole universe.[74]

This statement comes within a chapter in which different medical authorities have been offering different explanations about the causes of disease, much as in the Hippocratic treatises we find that one writer explained the fundamental forces to be fire and water, while another as air. Being the last explanation offered, and the most extensive, it seems intended to supersede the others, giving to *vāyu* a spiritual or divine dimension. Thus the fundamental cause of both disease and health is, for this authority, ultimately the disturbance or harmonious flowing of *vāyu*, the subtle vital principle, manifested as air.[75]

In the next passage, we again find a query about what this divine dimension has to do with medicine. The reply comes from Vāryovida, one of the sages taking part: "If a physician does not comprehend the vayu...how would he be able to forewarn a patient well in advance of its disastrous effects and how would he advise about the normal qualities of vāyu conducive to good health, improvement of strength and complexion, lustre, growth,

74. Ibid., vol. I 239.
75. On the significant similarities between ayurveda texts and *Breaths*, see Filliozat (1964) chapter 7.

attainment of knowledge and longevity?"[76] In other words, without this underpinning knowledge, how would the physician be able to go beyond the curing of disease to pro-actively helping his patient maintain optimal health and longevity, which is as much the aim of Āyurveda as the relief of suffering? These passages then indicate that the system aims at optimum well-being as much as the cure of specific diseases. Ideally the patient is expected to participate actively in his own recovery and maintenance of health verses 8-9) with the advice of the knowledgeable physician. Such an aim is also found in Sūtrasthāna I, verse 135: "Accomplishment of all objects ( i.e. actual prevention and cure of diseases) implies the proper application (of medicine). Success also implies the (presence of) the best physician endowed with all (good) qualities."[77]

Although such chapters and verses, which seem to ever strongly away from a rational approach in medicine, may represent what some have regarded as the Bhrāmaṇical overlay or later religious interpolations into the tradition,[78] they more likely reflect the very early association of physicians with the heterodox ascetics for whom spiritual liberation was the focus. Although most of the *Caraka* text discusses causes of disease and suffering in purely material, natural terms, these are put into a philosophical context. That the "theoretical" explanation was preserved suggests that it was important for the physicians. Such an association between ascetic philosophy and medicine enabled the physicians to place both the sufferings and the cures, and their own role and skills (which were the more immediate, daily facts of life of their art) into a much wider context. Moreover, it would encourage them to include examination of the wider context for the causal factors in disease. This is exactly the method which we find in *Caraka*.

While disturbance of the vital force, here *vāyu*, is recognised as the original cause of disease and misery, other more obvious and proximal causes, derived from this, form the greater part of *Caraka's* text. Among the most important of these are

---

76. Sharma and Dash (1994) vol. I 240.
77. Ibid., vol.I 61.
78. Zysk (1991) 30-35 and vs Chattopadhyaya (1979) 13, 179-188, 400-404.

unwholesome diet and imbalance of *doṣas*. Such causes are necessarily those dealt with on the practical daily level by the physician, and as such are given most prominence in the text. One such example is Sūtrasthāna IX, verse 4:

> Any disturbance in the equilibrium of *dhātus* (elements of the body) is known as disease and on the other hand the state of their equilibrium is health. Health and disease are also defined as pleasure and pain.[79]

## The Physician's Role, the Individual Patient's Role and the Self-healing Mechanism

"The four aspects of therapeutics are the physician, the medicament, the attendant and the patient." This statement begins the chapter on therapeutics of Sūtrasthāna IX. These four aspects are together responsible for the cure of diseases, provided they have the requisite qualities.[80] The physician should possess excellence in medical knowledge, extensive practical experience, dexterity and purity, critical approach, insight into other allied sciences, good memory, continued practice and reliance on an experienced preceptor.[81] Sūtrasthāna I, verse 133 re-reinforces this by saying,

> the wise one who aspires to be a physician should make special efforts to maintain his (good) qualities so he can be the life-giver to human beings.... It is only he who can relieve his patients of their ailments who is the best physician.[82]

The physician uses his knowledge and skill to choose the medicaments. (Sūtrasthāna I verse 120-123) The attendant and the patient play their part by carrying out faithfully the remedies given (IX, verses 8, 9). The quality of consciousness (inner mental state) of both the physician and the patient are important to the outcome.

Crucial to the physician's skill is first to understand the

79. Sharma and Dash, (1994), vol.I 184.
80. Ibid., 183.
81. Ibid., (verses 6, 21-23) 186, 189-190.
82. Ibid., 60-61.

patient's *prakṛti* (nature or individual mix of *doṣas*), then to ascertain which *doṣas* are out of balance. The out-of-balance state is the *vikṛti*. Next, by means of medicine, diet and other therapies, he helps to restore the balance within the whole context of the patient's life.

> One who knows the principles governing their correct application in consonance with the place, time and individual variation should be regarded as the best physician.[83]

Such treatment often opposes the excess or deficiency of the disequilibrium with things of opposite qualities. (Sūtrasthāna, I, 62-63). In this the physician is seen to be helping the body do what it naturally does.

A suggestion of this "natural homeostasis" is found in chapter XVI of Sūtrasthāna:

> the *dhātus* come to normalcy automatically irrespective of any external causative factor; that is to say both the imbalanced and balanced *dhātus* tend to fade away immediately after they are caused (verse 27).... By avoiding discordance-causing factors and adopting those responsible for the maintenance of equilibrium, discordance of *dhātus* is automatically prevented and their normal state of equilibrium is maintained. By taking recourse to concordant factors, the physician well-versed in treatment brings about equilibrium of *dhātus*.... (verses 34-38).[84]

As we have already seen such "factors" come from all aspects of a person's life: diet, environment, seasons, mind and emotions, lifestyle, exercise. In other words, the patient's life *as a whole* has to be taken into consideration.

Inherent in this approach is the understanding that there is a natural corrective mechanism within the body. The physician and the patient work with this process by two means: avoiding negative or disturbing factors while supplying positive or balancing ones. If this is done, the body automatically heals itself, or as the text puts it, re-establishes its equilibrium.

If we return to the Śārīrasthāna passage quoted above (V, 6-7) we also find that the passage suggests that although there are

83. Ibid., (verses 120-123), 59.
84. Ibid., 305, 307-308.

various proximal factors that bring on disease, ultimately what happens to a person is his own responsibility. This is according to the concepts of karma and of attachments to the world. Chapter I, verse 116-117 of Śārīrasthāna also states that

> the action performed in the previous life which is known as *daiva* (fate) also constitutes in due course causative factors for the manifestation of diseases.

Diseases due to such fate are not amenable to therapy and are curable "only after the results of past actions are exhausted."[85] While recognising the existence of such non-material factors in the cause of disease, ultimately for the physician, it is the frame of mind of the patient which is of crucial importance. Śārīrasthāna I, verse 132 states:

> But in the *context of the science of medicine* [emphasis mine], it is only the four-fold combination which is relevant as a causative factor of happiness and miseries (that is to say the wholesome combination is required to be adhered to and the unwholesome one to be given up for the maintenance of good health.)[86]

In another place, *Caraka* says,

> whatever act is done by one who is deranged of understanding, will or memory is to be regarded as a volitional transgression, *prajñāparādha* (an offence against nature or wisdom). It is the inducer of all pathological conditions.[87]

The spirit of this passage is similar with that of *The Art* XI quoted above (p. 60).

Śārīrasthāna, VI considers the subject of the human constitution or *prakṛti*. It is important to note that, as with the Greek use of nature, in *Caraka* the same word, *prakṛti*, is used for primordial nature, for nature in general and for the nature of the individual human body. Prose passage 4 states,

---

85. Ibid., vol. II, 340-341.
86. Ibid., 344.
87. Svoboda (1992) 155, translating Śārīrasthāna I, verses 102-108 [Sharma and Dash (1994) vol. II 337-338]. See also Sūtrasthāna XI, 56-63, which describes how people become vulnerable to disease producing situations by neglecting to care for the body.

> the body which is maintained in a state of equilibrium represents the conglomeration, *samudāya* of factors derived from the five *mahābhūtas* and this is the site of manifestation of consciousness.

To maintain a healthy state of equilibrium, not only are activities and foods conducive to it important, but also the right mental activities: i.e. right use of time, intellect and objects of senses (passage 8). As will be discussed in Chapter Four, each *doṣa* in the Ayurvedic system is related to particular mental–emotional predispositions inherent in a person's *prakṛti.* Aggravation of these mental–emotional states can be one of the factors that disturb the balance of the *doṣas,* setting the stage for disease in the body.

The results of this preliminary search for evidence of holistic characteristics in the Hippocratic *Corpus* and in *Caraka* has shown that both systems are deeply committed to this approach, indeed are constituted out of it. There are also differences between the two.

In *Caraka* the spiritual dimension is given greater prominence and is explicitly detailed, according to the tradition of the philosophical schools. This is perhaps because the social–religious climate in India at the time, while not totally unlike that of Greece, was different in that physicians had become less defensive about their craft, and were less concerned to distance themselves from heterodox ascetic traditions in healing, with which they shared common sources. In the Hippocratic *Corpus,* more explicit emphasis is given to the healing power of nature, and this is sensed as divine, but with few explicit references to spiritual factors.

In the Greek case, there is more evidence that the physicians were competing with other forms of healing (root doctors, root and charm sellers, temple medicine). They were concerned to defend the status of their profession and they were willing openly to debate the differing approaches with each other. While there are some examples of the physicians' awareness of mind–body–spirit interplay, this is given less attention relative to the text devoted to other subjects. However, if we take into account their conviction in the healing power of a divine nature, such interplay is implicit. In the *Corpus,* the theme of the physician as servant of nature's healing power is prominent. In *Caraka* we do not find such repeated references to prakṛti in this way.

The position of a "vital force" in the two traditions is comparable, if we accept the *Corpus*' implicit equation of it to nature's power. In *Breaths* this power of nature is identified with a specific element, air, present in the body as breath. Yet the fact that other authors do not mention this so directly, suggests that this was not a view held by all.

In *Caraka*, by contrast, definite prominence is given to *prāṇa* and its acceptance is assumed because the text has the appearance of homogeneity.

In many respects the two traditions are remarkably similar, as many of the earlier quotations reveal. Each recognises an inherent life principle, though different strands in the traditions may refer to it by different names. This principle is or partakes of the divine essence of creation. Each sees health as man's natural state based on balance—until circumstances or attitudes, beliefs, or emotions upset this equilibrium. Each sees the duty and skill of the physician to restore this natural balance by means which are readily to hand in nature, but which are applied with particular skill. They also recognise that the patient is responsible for and needs to be involved in this health-restoring process at all levels: body, mind and spirit. Each senses that ultimately it is the quality of consciousness that is the key factor in health and disease.

CHAPTER 3

# FOOD AND DIGESTION, HEALTH AND DISEASE

As we have seen in Chapter One, a key concept of holistic medicine is to take into consideration all aspects of a patient's life, both when assessing the nature of the illness or imbalance and in formulating the therapeutic strategy for restoring health and well-being. One of the major areas for consideration is the dietary habits of the patient. Holistic or natural medicine in modern Europe and in America has long emphasised the importance of diet in both the prevention of disease and as part of the treatment process. It is the very foundation of health.[1] In Britain, one osteopathic training institution is called the College of Osteopathy and Naturopathy. Naturopathy includes dietary regimes and fasting. Integral to Ayurvedic medicine, both past and present, is an emphasis on what constitutes a healthful diet for prevention and well-being, and methods of correcting the diet as part of treating illness. In recent years the phrase 'lifestyle' has become current in the language of health care, both conventional and complementary. It refers to the life habits of an individual in terms of his or her individual pattern of diet, exercise, recreation, work and relationships. As we shall see, the Hippocratic physicians also emphasised the importance of such factors as part of their attention to *bios* and *diaita*, the patient's mode of life.

'You are what you eat' became a catchphrase in the 1960s and 1970s as growth of the 'healthfood movement' accelerated.

---

1. See, for example, John Christopher, *The School of Natural Healing*; Jethro Kloss, *Back to Eden*; Henry Lindlahr, *Natural Therapeutics*; H.C.A Vogel, *The Nature Doctor*.

It captured the notion that what you eat literally forms you and has a major effect on how you feel, whether you are healthy or ill. This concept is in complete agreement with the author of *Ancient Medicine* III who attributes the origin of the art of medicine itself to diet. An examination of the ideas on diet and food in the Hippocratic treatises from a holistic, rather than a scholarly or medical science point of view reveals valuable sources for some of the ideas of holistic medicine on food and diet. In the texts there is present the strong conviction that food, diet and the process of transformation of food in the body is vitally important to health. Treatment of the patient through foods (and drinks) is fundamental in therapy. Given the influence of Hippocratic medicine until at least the sixteenth century, it is a likely primary source of this strong tradition in Western complementary medicine.

The Ayurvedic classical text, *Caraka Saṃhitā*, which is still being taught and practised today, similarly devotes a major part of its verses to aspects of diet in health and in illness. Its treatment protocols in use today comprise methods similar to those found in the *Corpus*.

## FOOD AND DIET IN THE *CORPUS*

Of the sixty treatises in the collection, no fewer than eight deal directly and largely with diet and food regimen: *Nutriment, Regimen I-IV, Regimen in Acute Diseases* with its Appendix, *Regimen in Health*. Others, such as *Humours, Aphorisms*, the three books of *Diseases, Internal Affections* and the seven books of *Epidemics* mention diet and food as part of treatment. In addition, *Ancient Medicine*, while not having food or diet in its title in a large part argues that diet and treatment of disease through diet is actually the origin and main craft of medicine. Hippocratic texts on gynaecology, embryology, and the origins of man, are also interested in nutrition, especially as regards the formation and nourishment of the embryo. They treat food and diet as being directly linked to healthy or problematic conceptions, pregnancies, and their treatment. The author of *Nature of Man* IX cites regimen as one of the two causes of disease, the other being air.

We have seen when examining the philosophical background to the Hippocratic authors that they shared earlier ideas about the creation and constitution of the world from fundamental elements that exist in the body, ideally balanced in a state of harmony through being blended and compounded together, *krasis*, so that no single element stands alone, isolated. Being separate and uncompounded means the element becomes too powerful or strong and dominates the others, *monarchia*. The Hippocratic physicians applied these ideas to their understanding of diseases caused by harmful diet and in their treatment of acute, feverish diseases, as well as to their programmes for health maintenance.

## Concepts of Food and Digestion

From this common pool of ideas, each Hippocratic author often developed his own idiosyncratic approach. For example, evidently influenced not only by Heraclitus, but also Empedocles, and Anaxagoras,[2] the author of *Regimen I* emphasises fire and water as his elements or humours, and describes the origin of male and female difference in terms of a preponderance of heat-dryness or cold-moistness taken from food stuffs. Thus females naturally "grow from food, drinks and pursuits that are cold, moist and gentle" (XXVII). That he considers digestion crucial to ongoing life is shown by his powerful, poetic description of the belly as the source of nutrition, growth and health in the body, sorting what is beneficial for the body from what is not.

> The belly is made the greatest, a steward for dry water and moist, to give to all and to take from all, the power of the sea, nurse of creatures suited to it destroyer of those not suited ... a copy of the earth, which alters all things that fall into it (X).[3]

In chapter IX he describes how the various tissues of the body are formed through the action of fire, water, and movement:

> The fire, meanwhile, being moved out of the moisture which was mixed with it, arranges the body according to nature

2. Jones (1979) vol. IV xliii.
3. Ibid., 247.

> through the following necessity. Through the hard and dry parts it cannot make itself lasting passages, because it has no nourishment; but it can through the moist and soft, for these are its nourishment. Yet in these too there is dryness not consumed by the fire, and these dry parts become compacted one with another. So the fire shut up in the innermost part both is most abundant and made for itself the greatest passage. For there the moisture was most abundant, and it is called the belly. There from the fire burst forth, since it had no nourishment and made passages for the breath and to supply and distribute nourishment. The fire shut up in the rest of the body made itself three passages, the moistest part of the fire being in those places called the hollow veins. And in the middle of these that which remains of the water becomes compacted and congeals. It is called flesh.[4]

The author sums up the whole approach of the Hippocratic to diet, health and disease in the following account:

> I maintain that he who aspires to treat correctly of human regimen must first acquire knowledge and discernment of the nature of man in general knowledge of its primary constituents and discernment of the components by which it is controlled [i.e. for him fire and water] These things the author must know, and further the power possessed severally by all the foods, and drinks of our regimen, both the power each of them possessed by nature and the power given them by the constraint of human art. For it is necessary to know both how one ought to lessen the power of these when they are strong by nature, and when they are weak to add by art strength to them, seizing each opportunity as it occurs...eating alone will not keep a man well; he must also take exercise. For food and exercise, while possessing opposite qualities, yet work together to produce health....If it were possible to discover for the constitution of each individual a due proportion of food to exercise, with no

4. Ibid., 245, 247.

> inaccuracy either of excess or of defect, an exact discovery of health for men would have been made. [although this perfect knowledge is not possible since the physician cannot watch the person all the time]...if there occur even a small deficiency of one or the other, in the course of time the body must be overpowered by the excess and fall sick.... For diseases do not arise among men all at once; they gather themselves together gradually before appearing with a sudden spring. So I have discovered the symptoms shown in a patient before health is mastered by disease, and how these are to be replaced by a state of health.[5]

In XXXV-XXXVI, the author even relates diet and regimen, based on the blending of fire and water, to the health of the soul itself:

> It is blending then [of fire-water, dry-moist] that is as I have now explained, the cause of the soul's intelligence or want of it; regimen can make this blending either better or worse.

(He does, however, go on to say that regimen and blending cannot moderate every aspect of the person, the exceptions being "irascibility, indolence, craftiness, simplicity, quarrelsomeness and benevolence" (XXXVI).[6]

We find in the above the main themes of the Hippocratic medicine concerning diet, health and disease: (1) harmony/*harmonia*, balance and blending/*krasis* among the elements, or humours, or sometimes simply 'powers'/*dunameis*; (2) the nature of the nutritive process; (3) the idea of surfeit and depletion; (4) the relationship between diet and exercise and between diet, exercise and disease; (5) the relationship between food and mental-emotional states; and (6) the blending of foods' powers which occurs in the digestive organs, both naturally and, when needed, by the physician's art and special reasoning, *logismos*. *Logismos* reveals how the body functions and the individual patient's nature or blend of humours relate to his environment. Specific treatment with emetics and purging herbs to influence the internal environment of the alimentary canal are

5. Ibid., 227-231.
6. Ibid., 293.

not mentioned in this quote from *Regimen I*, but do accompany dietary treatment in the other works.

We find echoes and further details of these themes in the other writers on medicine. *Ancient Medicine* also emphasises knowledge of diet and nutrition as the essential art of medicine. It is necessary to know not only the strengths of foods but also how to render them less powerful by *krasis*, blending and compounding. For this author, however, the elements are not heat-cold, dry-moist, but rather 'powers' or qualities, especially the powers of tastes: acid, acrid, astringent, bitter, pungent. Also important are the effects of these when in excess or deficiency.

*Regimen in Acute Diseases* gives details of how to apply these ideas of food qualities to acute feverish diseases. *Regimen in Health* focuses on the optimum health of the individual gained by relating food and diet to the individual constitution. *Regimen III* focuses on the balance between diet and exercise. *Regimen II* is concerned to detail the qualities of different foods. *Regimen IV* approaches disease through the understanding of dreams but the prescriptions are those of special diet and exercises, purges and emetics. In *Diseases I-III* we have details of the application of dietary methods, along with herbal (drug) therapy, to various specific diseases, some of which we can recognize, such as pneumonia. *Diseases IV* cites the four humours—blood, phlegm, yellow bile and black bile—as the elements to be balanced. *Diseases of Women* cites no theoretical considerations but does choose foods on the basis of whether they promote health for the mother, seed, or embryo via their moistening-drying qualities. *Epidemics I* and 2 mentions few if any details of treatment in its description of the main diseases in a locality and its individual case histories, but as Jones has pointed out, "the writer assumes that the usual methods were followed...",[7] i.e. those outlined in, for example, *Regimen in Acute Diseases*: diet and herbs to influence the digestive system and thus the body as a whole.

Having identified the main themes of the dietary approach of the Hippocratic physicians we can now look at their concepts in

---

7. Jones (1972) vol. I xviii-xix.

more detail. We are struck first by the image of foods being cooked in a container that serves as the metaphor for what is central to these themes: the process of digestion and the nutrition of the body. Their ideas about these processes consist in what may be called primary and secondary aspects, plus the pathological effects when the process is imbalanced, for which they prescribe remedies using special foods and cleansing techniques along with exercise or rest.

## Metaphor and Substance, Fire and Food in the Cooking Pot

The story of Prometheus stealing fire from the gods in order to help humanity preserves for us the importance to the ancient Greeks of fire to human survival. This centrality is reiterated in the Hippocratic treatises through the metaphor of *pepsis.* Jones renders this word as 'coction', a term somewhat remote to us today and which perhaps can be more familiarly taken as simply 'cooking'. To understand how the ancient Greeks understood this word we can refer to a Greek lexicon which reveals that the root word is *pesso* which has several nuances of meaning. It can mean to soften, as in the sun which softens and thereby ripens fruit; to boil, and generally to cook, also to bake; it can mean to digest. In a metaphorical sense it was also used to mean to 'stomach' or 'digest' an experience, and even to nurse and, interestingly, to heal as of a wound.[8]

When physician-writers of the *Corpus* chose the word *pepsis* to describe the processes of transformation which take place in the body, such nuances of meaning may all be implied. They used the term not only in its strict sense relating to the digestion (transformation) of food, but also to the sense relating to other transformations in the body, particularly the changes in the various secretions and discharges produced by the body—the humours, and even to bodily tissues themselves—the flesh.[9]

Perhaps the best description of coction in the *Corpus*, as Jones has pointed out, is found in *Ancient Medicine*, chapters XVIII

8. Liddell and Scott 556.
9. For more on this see Chapter Four. A humour or sometimes a tissue is either 'concocted', a state of health, or 'unconcocted', a pathological or unbalanced state.

and XIX. [It is] "the most complete account of coction as the ancient physiologists conceived of it. It is really the process that leads to *krasis* as result...an action which so combines the opposing humours that there results a perfect fusion of all. No one is left in excess so as to cause trouble or pain to the human individual. The writer takes three types of illnesses— the common cold, ophthalmia, and pneumonia—and shows that as they grow better the discharges become less acid and thicker as a result of *pepsis*."[10] In these chapters the process is described regarding deranged humour (the discharges), but elsewhere in the work the author also uses it to apply to the processing of foods as well. Throughout the *Corpus* the 'processing' of both foods and humours in the body and the action of herbs to influence these, are closely connected.

Another description of coction, epitomising the ancient view of the world which saw a unity in all natural processes, is found in *Airs, Waters, Places*, VIII. Speaking of waters, but relating them to the entire microcosm-macrocosm he says:

> Not only from pools does the sun raise this part, but from sea and from whatever has moisture in it—and there is moisture in everything. Even from men it raises the finest and lightest part of their juices...[and from moisture in clouds, the sun's power means] the lightest part of it remains and is sweetened as the heat of the sun produces coction, just as all other things become sweeter through coction.[11]

## Primary Digestion: The Transformation and Assimilation of Food to Nourish Bodily Tissues

Thorough digestion and assimilation of foodstuffs is held to be of great importance by the writers on diet, for any impairment of the process of proper nourishment upsets balance and sets the stage for disease. The subject is looked at from various viewpoints. In *Ancient Medicine* foods that are themselves uncompounded[12]

---

10. Jones (1972) vol.I li.
11. Jones (1972) vol.I 91.
12. For example, Jones (1972) vol. I 38, *akretos*.

and are therefore too 'strong' are not healthful for the body. They are considered difficult to digest, to breakdown and transform, in other words, to cook and blend with others and therefore they cannot be fully assimilated to tissues. They are thus capable of causing injury or disease by initiating imbalance. Disease can be caused by either too much or too little food;[13] by either depletion or unseasonable repletion;[14] or by prompting the separation of secretions which, being thus isolated or uncompounded cause disorder.[15] In chapter IX it is recognised that depletion produces as many ills as repletion.[16]

For the writer of *Regimen in Acute Diseases*, sudden changes in eating habits are the crucial factor (XXXI).[17] In *Regimen III* we find the idea that digestion can be overwhelmed by an excess of exercise which impairs nourishment, or by excess food which overwhelms the digestion and thus the body (LXVII).[18] Seasonal and constitutional factors as well as age and even sex are also taken into account (XXXII).[19]

The process of cooking is implied in the idea of digestion and thus the idea of some kind of fire or heat as fuel to the transformation process. Inside the body this catalyst is supplied by the

---

13. Ibid., 27.
14. Ibid., 29 *akairou*.
15. Ibid., 38 *apokrithe*, *akretos*, *tarachos*. See also chapter III.
16. Ibid., 27.
17. Jones (1981) vol. II 89 and especially XXXV: "the chief causes of diseases are the most violent changes in what concerns our consitutions and habits." 91.
18. Jones (1979) vol. IV 367: "the discovery I have made is how to diagnose what is the overpowering element in the body, whether exercises overpower food or food overpowers exercises; how to cure each excess and to ensure good health so as to prevent the approach of disease, unless very serious and many blunders be made. In such cases there is the need of drugs while in some there are that not even drugs can cure."
19. Ibid., 275: "Such bodies as are blended of the strongest fire and the densest water turn out strong and robust physically, but need great caution. For they are subject to great changes in either direction and fall into illness at the onset of the water and likewise at those of the fire. Accordingly it is beneficial for a man of this type to counteract the seasons of the year in the diet he follows, employing one inclined to fire when the onset of water occurs, and one inclined to water when the onset of fire occurs, changing it gradually as the season itself changes."

body's innate heat.[20] Also implicit is the idea of some fluid aspect, for it was recognized that the stomach contains fluids and that food is changed into a fluid form in the stomach. *Nutriment* LV states that "moisture is the vehicle of nutriment".[21] There is also some recognition that air is necessary to, or at least concomitant with the process.

Thus we have the everyday observation of food transformed by cooking used to describe the inner process of digestion, the essentials of which are fire (the innate heat), the cooking pot (body or stomach) which contains the variety of food eaten and also a liquid medium in which the food is 'cooked' (moisture). When any aspect of this digestive/cooking process is disturbed, the way is paved for the body's balance to be upset and disease conditions to occur.

A feature of this cooking process, whether internal or external, is that of *krasis.* In the writings, foods are often described in terms of their strengths. This is a particular theme in *Ancient Medicine.* By strength is understood the strength of any particular quality of the food, for example its moistness, dryness, hardness (or crudeness),

20. *thermos*. We do not find much reference to the idea of innate heat in the Hippocratic *Corpus*, although it is a feature of the thought of previous or contemporary writers who took an interest in the body. (e.g. Empedocles, Aristotle, Plato) It was recognised to be a vital element of the body, necessary for life. In the *Corpus* statements about it are rather inferred from statements on the dangers of cold. (*Aphorisms* I and XIV; *Regimen* III, LXXIX; *Regimen In Health* VII) *Nutriment* explains that the lungs draw 'a nourishment' ( i.e. air) to cool the 'opposite of that of the body' i.e. the innate heat (XXIX). (The idea is to prevent the heat that is seated in the heart, from becoming too extreme.); and that "Root of veins, liver, root of arteries, heart. Out of these travel to all parts blood and breath, and heat/*thermasin* passes through them"(XXXI). Fleshes does call *thermos* 'immortal' and the agent of transformations in the cosmos and the body (Potter (1995) vol. VIII, 133-135, 147,ff.) However, as Jones has pointed out, though the author of *Ancient Medicine* is concerned to promote the idea that disease and health have little to do with 'the hot', or 'the cold' he would agree that heat is a necessary concomitant of the digestive process. (He is opposed to the attribution of health or disease to the actions of heat and cold, because his method of medicine is based on mixing and blending through pepsis of foods and tastes) But, as Jones states, both the heat of digestion and the consequential heating of the body by this process "must have coloured the notion of pepsis as generally held" And the concept of innate heat "was thought to have a powerful influence upon the bodily functions." Jones (1972) vol. I, li-lii.
21. Jones (1972) vol. I 361.

cold or heat and other qualities of foods. Such strength is also understood to be relative to the individual, for example whether he is physically weak or strong, whether he or she habitually eats one or two meals a day, or whether he is of a moist or dry constitution (*Regimen in Acute Diseases,* XXXVII). Although some foods are so strong and crude as to not be worth the trouble, many strong foods can be rendered acceptable and nourishing to the body by being cooked in certain ways. For example, boiling adds moisture to dry foods, baking makes inherently moist foods less moist and more dry. Barley, which is inherently moist and cooling, when made into cakes becomes drier than barley gruel. In other cases foods of differing strengths and qualities may be cooked together, thereby modifying and moderating their individual properties. The result is a congenial and milder, therefore more nutritious and assimilable whole.

This aspect of cooking is captured in the term *krasis,* meaning a blending, mixing or compounding. *Krasis* occurs naturally during the inner digestion as well as during preparatory cooking, and it can be influenced directly by special preparations of foods and drugs.

The physician is one who has studied and gathered knowledge about these natural healthful processes and can advise people on which foods are suitable or unsuitable for each individual's optimum health. He is also the one who knows what foods to administer or withhold in disease. (Therapeutic fasting is an important method of the physician's repertoire of skills.) As we have just seen, he also knows how to transform foods to moderate their qualities so that they are helpful and less dangerous to the body. This skill is basically a more specialized form of cooking: the art of changing foods' qualities by cooking them in various ways, and with other foods of different qualities. In this sense the physician has also to be himself a master of the arts of *pepsis* and *krasis*: cooking and mixing, blending, compounding.[22]

22. With respect, I must here disagree with Elizbeth Craik (Wilkins, et al., 1995), 349 when she says the Hippocratics had little first-hand knowledge of cooking.

Cooking and the proper preparation of food was considered so important it ranks as an important skill in the physicians' arts, or crafts, of medicine. The authors of *Regimen I* and *II* agree with the author of *Ancient Medicine*, for in their treatises we find that the physician himself must know the arts of cooking or coction of food. We have quoted from *Regimen I* above that the powers of foods could be "constrained by human art". *Regimen II* similarly discusses the "power of various foods and drinks, both what they are by nature and by *art*" (emphasis mine) (XXXI), in other words, how they can be modified by the physician's specialized skill. The powers mentioned are sometimes qualities of heat/cold, moist/dry; sometimes what we would call effects, such as binding, laxative, astringent, diuretic; sometimes they are tastes, such as astringency, salty, insipid, pungent, acrid, sweet; sometimes they are type of food such as fatty, oily. Both by mixing them with substances of opposite qualities and by cooking them in special ways the physicians achieve the moderation and mildness conducive to complete digestion and assimilation. They could modify foods that were 'too strong' or which, in a particular body, became too strong and therefore separated and dominant.

For example, *Ancient Medicine* describes some foods as being too strong and therefore creating harm: in the past "many and terrible were the sufferings of men from strong and brutish living when they partook of crude foods, uncompounded and possessing great powers".[23] Indeed the discovery of how to change strong foods to be more digestible is the very art of medicine.

> For this reason too the ancients seem to me to have sought for nourishment that harmonised with their constitution,

---

methods. If by this term she means cooking as a culinary art as we understand it today for the primary purpose of pleasure, she may be right. But that the physicians believed they needed to know the *techne* of choosing foods based on their tastes and other qualities and the different methods of cooking foods to balance them is most in evidence in the *Corpus*. In *Regimen II* we have many details of the effects of different foods and herbs on the body, along with their tastes and qualities. This may seem an 'austere' approach to us but it was an important part of their professional skills.

23. Jones (1972) vol. I 19-20.

> and to have discovered that which we use now. So from wheat, after steeping it, winnowing, grinding and sifting, kneading, baking, they produced bread, and from barley they produced cake. Experimenting with food they boiled or baked, after mixing, many other things, combining the strong and uncompounded with the weaker components so as to adapt all to the constitution and power of man, thinking that from foods which, being too strong, the human constitution cannot assimilate when eaten, will come pain, disease, and death, while from such as can be assimilated will come nourishment, growth, and health. To this discovery and research what juster or more appropriate name could be given than medicine, seeing that it has been discovered with a view to the health, saving and nourishment of man, in the place of that mode of living from which came the pain, disease and death?[24]

He continues (VI):

> all the causes of pain can be reduced to one, namely, it is the strongest foods that hurt a man most and most obviously, whether he be well or ill.[25]

Hence the need, as discussed previously, to moderate food by various methods, e.g. grinding and cooking, along with mixing and blending it with other foods, and presumably herbs, to create a new food which can be accepted, digested and assimilated and therefore nourish the body tissues.

The author of *Regimen II* agrees, saying:

> The powers of food severally ought to be diminished or increased in the following way, as it is known that out of fire and water are composed all things, both animal and vegetable, and that through them all things grow and into them they are dissolved. Take away their power from strong foods by boiling and cooling many times; remove moisture from moist things by grilling and roasting them; soak and

24. Ibid.
25. Ibid., 23.

> moisten dry things, soak and boil salt things, bitter and sharp things mix with sweet, and astringent things mix with oily.... Foods grilled or roasted are more binding than raw, because the fire has taken away the moisture, the juice and the fat. So when they fall into the belly they drag to themselves the moisture from the belly, burning up the mouths of the veins, drying and heating them so as to shut up the passages for liquids.... Accordingly it is necessary to know the property, not only of foods themselves, whether of corn, drink or meat, but also of the country from which they come (LVI).[26]

Knowledge of how diet and cooking methods can be refined to correspond to individual constitutions is also important and is attested in several of the treatises. *Regimen II* relates different dietary treatments to different kinds of individuals, though constitutions in terms of the four humours are not mentioned, only in terms of moistness and dryness, heat and cold. He then goes on to "show what power each one has in particular" (XXXIX), in subsequent chapters detailing very many foods and drinks according to whether they—or more precisely their effects on the human body—are drying or moistening, warming or cooling, or laxative, binding or astringent, or diuretic. He also discusses how to cook them to balance their powers.[27] The foods include various cereals, meats, eggs and cheeses, vegetables and fruits, wines and vinegars and honey.

*Regimen in Acute Diseases* focuses mainly on the therapeutic properties of barley gruel for acute diseases, but also describes various kinds of wines, vinegars, hydromels (water and honey), oxymels (vinegar and honey) according to their effects on individual bodies. Used in this therapeutic way such foodstuffs become in effect medicines. *Regimen II* canvasses many foods and drinks and describes them according to their qualities. The foods, including animals, fish, as well as vegetable and dairy products, are described in terms of their qualities: heat-cold,

26. Jones (1979) vol. IV 337-339.
27. The first item on the list interestingly is barley, because it was the staple cereal in Greece, and so, as we shall see below, an important food for the Hippocratic physician.

moisture-dryness, heaviness-lightness. Interestingly, whether they pass easily by stool and urine is also described. Thus proper elimination of waste products created by a certain food is seen to be an important factor. The qualities of some foods may be moderated by special cooking methods or by mixing with other foods. For example,

> millet groats and husk are dry and binding; with figs they are strong nourishment for hard workers. Whole millet by itself boiled is nourishing but it does not pass by stool (XLV).[28]

*Regimen I*, as discussed above (p. 4-7), relates different constitutional types, *phuseis*, in terms of their varying blend of fire and water to diet, exercise, age, and environmental factors (seasons) and prescribes regimen accordingly. Though coction is not mentioned, disease is said to be caused by either an imbalance between diet and exercise or imbalance in the blend of fire and water (including dryness, moisture, heat and cold) in the body, one becoming dominant. Fire seems to be the vehicle of the transformations, as it is responsible for movement. Disease is overcome and health restored through mixing again, which restores harmony (II, III, IV, VIII,XXXII).[29]

The author of *Ancient Medicine* certainly considered such skills to be the mainstay of medicine:

> Accordingly there could surely be nothing more useful or more necessary to know than these things, and how the first discoverers, pursuing their inquiries excellently and with suitable application of reason to the nature of man, made their discoveries and thought the art worthy to be ascribed to a god (XIV).... Since this at least I think a

28. Jones (1979) vol. IV 315-317. See also 307-315.
29. Ibid., 231-233, 243, and 275. *diakrenomena and symmisgomena* (234) (As well as practical instruction, this treatise has a large proportion of what seems to be a mystical approach to the nature of man, recalling Alcmaeon, Anaxagoras, Pythogoras and Empedocles!) Compare *Ancient Medicine*, XVIII: "when the evil comes from cold alone, unaccompanied by anything else, there is always the some change, heat following chill and chill heat...in all other instances where acrid and unmixed humours come into play, I am confident that the cause is the same, and that restoration results from coction and mixture." Jones (1972), vol. I, 47-49.

physician must know and be at great pains to know, about natural science, if he is going to perform aught of his duty, what a man is in relation to foods and drinks, and to habits generally and what will be the effects of each on each individual (XX).[30]

The author of *Regimen I*, having stated in chapter XV that "In other respects too nature is the same as the physician's art", goes on to state in chapter XVII:

Builders out of diverse materials fashion a harmony, moistening what is dry, drying what is moist, dividing wholes and putting together what is divided.... It is a copy of the diet of man, moistening the dry, drying the moist, they divide wholes and put together what is divided. All these being diverse are harmonious (XVII).

Cooks are responsible for preparing for men dishes of ingredients that disagree while agreeing, mixing together things of all sorts, from things that are the same, things that are not the same to be food and drink for a man (XVIII).

The finest water and the rarest fire, on being blended together in the human body, produce the most healthy condition (XXXII).[31]

A specific example of this skill is found in *Regimen* II, LVI, quoted previously (p. 95-96).

Another way that food can create imbalance is if it is not proportionate to exercise. *Regimen III* is chiefly concerned to balance diet with exercise: the one nourishes and builds up the body, the other reduces it; both are needed, so that one does not overpower the other. This, he says, is his great 'discovery'. Accordingly, in treating disease, he recommends specific diets or exercise which restore any imbalance of harmony between the two. The term 'diets' here is also understood to include such

30. Jones (1972) vol. I 37, 53-54.
31. Jones (1979) vol. IV 255, 257, 273 (*Hudatos de to leptotaton kai puros to araiotaton*). Jones comments, "The great importance attached to regimen in this treatise is characteristic of all that is best in Greek medicine. Upon it the physician relied, both to preserve health and to heal diseases" (xlvii).

treatments as purgings and emetics which restore the internal digestive environment to balance. This author also takes account of the seasons, geography (similar to the author of *Airs, Waters and Places*), the person's individual nature or constitution (including age), and the qualities of different foods and exercises when prescribing either diet or exercise. Thus he states:

> First the constitutions of men differ; dry constitutions for instance, are more or less dry as compared with themselves or as compared with one another.... The various ages have different needs. Moreover the different districts, the shifting of the winds, the changes of the seasons, the constitutions of the year. Foods themselves exhibit many differences.[32]

The author of *Regimen in Health*, though he doesn't set out to theorise about health and disease as such, makes his prescriptions for the healthy layman along similar lines, i.e., according to individual nature and other factors. He states for example, in chapter II:

> Those with physiques that are fleshy, soft and red find it beneficial to adopt a rather dry regimen for the greater part of the year. For the nature of these physiques is moist. Those that are lean and sinewy, whether ruddy or dark, should adopt a moister regimen for the greater part of the time for the bodies of such are constitutionally dry.[33]

For this author and for the author of *Regimen III* emetics and clysters (enemas) are not only used in the presence of disease but also as part of a health maintenance regime. Thus, in chapter V, he states:

> Use emetics during the six winter months, for this period engenders more phlegm than does the summer and in it occur the diseases that attack the head and the region above the diaphragm. But when the weather is hot, use clysters, for the season is burning, the body bilious, heaviness is

32. Ibid., 367.
33. Ibid., 47, 46 *eidesi* for physiques, *phusis* for nature.

> felt in the loins and knees...so the body must be cooled and the humours that rise must be drawn downwards from these regions.[34]

Evidently it was quite common for people to live according to such regimes, for he also states:.

> He who is in the habit of taking an emetic twice a month will find it better to do so on two successive days than once every fortnight, the usual custom is just the contrary.[35]

The purpose of the above treatments was either to keep the elements in harmony (defined as blended) or to restore harmony if they become imbalanced through diet. This then is the sort of knowledge the physician would need to know in order to prescribe the foods and cooking methods needed for a sick patient. The physician's role is not to be concerned with the pleasurable aspect of food consumption, but to be concerned with the healthful aspect, being convinced that, as the author of *Regimen in Health* says, "A wise man should consider that health is the greatest of human blessings, and learn how by his own thought to derive benefit in his illness" (IX).[36] If diseases could be caused by imbalance in foods consumed or in the digestive process of foods inside the body, the physician's *techne* would consist in redressing the balance by prescribing foods which, through their qualities and the way they were prepared, would reinstate good digestion and re-constitute the body in a sound or healthy state.

## Secondary or "Sequential Digestion"

We mentioned earlier that innate heat was recognized to be necessary for the digestive-nutritive process. In the body's

34. Ibid., 51.
35. Ibid., 53. Edelstein in "the Dietetics of Antiquity" (*Ancient Medicine*, 304-305) has said that such attention to bodily health must have been the prerogative of the leisured classes only. However, as Phillips points out (*Greek Medicine*, 19), Herodotus had commented that the Egyptians were in the habit of taking purgings regularly and "they were the healthiest of peoples". Similarly today in India quite ordinary people know the value and practice of cleansing procedures such as fasting and taking enemas and emetics, so it is not beyond the realm of possibility that the case was so in ancient Greece.
36. Ibid., 59. Compare with view of *Ancient Medicine*, cf. Chapter Two, 619 above.

digestive tract this is supplied by the body's own heat. The concept of 'innate heat' was held by many thinkers and writers of the period to be essentially related to, and sometimes the equivalent of that life principle discussed by the presocratic philosophers. Parmenides correlated cold with death and warmth with life, and Empedocles and Alcmaeon developed this idea further.[37] According to Longrigg, "it was widely adopted by the Hippocratic writers and subsequently taken up by Philistion, Plato and Aristotle."[38] There are several instances in the treatises where signs that indicate a turn for the worse, or imminent death in the acute fever cases occur when the extremities are cold. It is also recognized that it is possible for the body to become too hot. Indeed one of the functions of respiration is to cool or moderate the innate heat, according to Empedocles and, later, Philistion.[39] From this we can see that innate heat, like air, is a physical aspect or manifestation of the life-giving, life-sustaining, divine Vital Force. At the level of bodily substance, another manifestation is that of blood. For the Hippocratic physician the creation of and maintenance of good quality blood was an important aspect of health. How did he view its creation?

Longrigg has pointed out that the natural warmth of the body is also the "agent of embryological, digestive and other physiological processes,"[40] primarily through the idea of coction or cooking. He has shown that originally the idea of heat breaking down nutriment was described as one of "putrefaction, or sepsis, by Empedocles. But by the time we encounter it in the Hippocratic *Corpus* and Aristotle it has changed to one of *pepsis* (softening, ripening, maturing, cooking)."[41]

According to Empedocles, after digestion, the next stage is the formation of blood. Once food is digested, the resultant substance, the nutriment, forms blood and it is blood which goes on to nourish tissues by a continuing process of *pepsis.*

---

37. Longrigg (1993) 73. Parmenides' ideas are preserved in Theophrastus' *De sensibus*, D.K. 64A28.
38. Ibid.
39. Ibid.
40. Ibid., 98.
41. Ibid., 74.

According to Simplicius, Longrigg shows, nutriment goes from the stomach to the liver where it is turned into [i.e., further transformed or 'digested'] blood. Thus blood is the 'agent of nutrition.'

The ideas of Empedocles found expression in the medical corpus. *Ancient Medicine*, XXII expresses these ideas when it states that the normal functions of the liver and spleen are to 'digest and discharge'.

Empedocles considered breast milk to be a surplus residue of blood, a bodily substance formed from the ongoing 'digestion' of blood tissue. Diogenes said that blood is 'consumed' by the fleshy parts, again using a metaphor of eating and digestion: it nourishes them or is transformed into them. Diogenes also believes that semen is surplus nutriment, i.e. blood, because blood is 'concocted' by the superior innate heat of the male.[42] The vital air or *pneuma* mixed with it gave it its frothy appearance. Longrigg goes on to say that this series of sequential digestive processes via coction, beginning with blood and ending in either breastmilk or semen, "was to prove highly influential in the history of biology. It was adopted by Aristotle,...later adopted by...Herophilus and Erasistratus ...[and] also taken over by the Stoics and Galen subsequently subscribed to it."[43]

Among the Hippocratics we find the same ideas. Interestingly in *Nutriment*, VII, the author states that

> power of nutriment reaches to bone and to all the parts of bone, to sinew, to vein, to artery, to muscle, to membrane, to flesh, fat, bone, phlegm, marrow, brain, spinal marrow, the intestines and all their parts; it also reaches to heat, breath and moisture.

This in itself may not be the same as saying these are formed via sequential digestion but in chapter LI-LII we find

> Pus comes from flesh; pus-like lymph comes from blood and moisture generally. Pus is nutriment for a sore, lymph is nutriment for a vein and artery. Marrow nutriment of bone, and through this a callous forms.[44]

42. Ibid., 79, 80.
43. Ibid., 80.
44. Jones (1972) vol.I 345, 361.

These statements indicate that the physician-writer did envisage some parts of the body nourishing and making possible the formation of other parts, a form of sequential digestion and nourishment.

The final tissue named in the list just quoted is the bone marrow. Marrow appears to have been a very special tissue for the Hippocratic physicians. In the treatises dealing with the formation of the body parts or with generation and embryology (*Fleshes, On Generation, The Nature of the Child*) we find an interest in this tissue. It begins in the brain and fills the spine, hence, spinal fluid – bone marrow, but permeates "the loins and the whole body" and is the vehicle for the sperm to reach the penis.[45] Marrow seems to contain, in a way different from the blood, an essence of the creative life-force in the body, the life-force that empowers the generation of offspring, that makes fertility possible.[46] There are parallels for this bodily product in the concept of *ojas* in Ayurvedic medicine, as will be discussed later.

Apart from *Nutriment, Fleshes* also describes the formation of different tissues through the action of heat and even in terms of cooking. Thus the hollow vessels, throat, gullet, stomach and intestines are formed by the warming, drying, and hardening of a moist, cold or glutinous substance by heat. Though not stated, presumably the vehicle for this heat is the blood.

For several of the Hippocratic physicians, blood, a fluid medium partaking of vital air and heat, is the 'agent of nutrition'. It goes on to be transformed via a process described in terms related to consumption, nutriment and digestion into the other tissues of the body.

## Ideas about the Powers of Tastes

One aspect of the herbal medicine found in *Caraka* is the classification of drugs and foods according not only to the pairs of opposites (moist-dry, heating-cooling), but also according to taste. It is worth investigating if this tradition is also found in Hippocratic medicine.

---

45. Lonie (1981) 1-2.
46. Alcmaeon said that semen comes from brain and from marrow. In the Timaeus, spinal marrow is called the universal 'seed-stuff' (Phillips (1973) 124-125).

We do not find a great deal of discussion about tastes in the treatises on diet, as compared with discussions of constitutions, seasons, humours; but there is some. The writer of *Ancient Medicine*, while criticising other physicians for basing their medicine on irrelevant hypotheses that heat and cold cause disease in the body (after Empedocles), himself seems to put forward the idea that certain tastes—and whether or not they are too strong, or remain properly blended and digested—are the basic factors in the effects we see in the body. The tastes of acid, bitter, acrid, pungent are cited as the main factors in illness.

> For each of these differences produces in a human being an effect and a change of one sort or another, and upon these differences is based all the dieting of a man, whether he be in health, recovering from an illness or suffering from one.... For they [the ancient originators of medicine] did not consider that the dry or the moist or the hot or the cold or anything else of the kind injures a man, or that he has need of any such thing, but they considered that it is the strength of each thing, that which being too powerful for the human constitution, it cannot assimilate, which causes harms, and this they sought to take away. The strongest part of the sweet is the sweetest, of the bitter, the most bitter, of the acid the most acid and each of all the component parts of man has its extreme. For these they saw are component parts of man, and that they are injurious to him; for there is in man salt and bitter, sweet and acid, astringent and insipid and a vast number of other things possessing properties of all sorts, both in strength and number.... Moreover, of the foods that are unsuitable for us and hurt a man when taken, each one of them is either bitter, or salty, or acidic or something else uncompounded and strong, and for this reason we are disordered by them, just as were are by the secretions separated off in the body.[47]

---

47. Jones (1972) vol. I 37-39.

Chapter XV continues

> For it is not the heat which possesses the great power, but the astringent and the insipid and the other qualities I have mentioned, both in man and out of man, whether eaten or drunk, whether applied externally as ointment or as plaster.[48]

Chapter XVII continues

> men are not feverish merely through heat...the truth being that one and the same thing is both bitter and hot or acid and hot or salt and hot.... It is these things [e.g. the tastes] which cause the harm. Heat is present but merely as a concomitant.[49]

In *Ancient Medicine,* XIX, the disturbing humours, ('humour' evidently here meaning any fluid discharge, such as that from the eyes) are also identified in terms of the tastes, i.e., acrid etc., suggesting that assessments of bodily fluid secretions (humours) were made according to their tastes. Taste is also an indicator of coction. Thus discharges settling in the eyes are said to be acrid until concocted while discharges settling in the throat are salty until concocted. Yellow bile and nausea are related to the bitter principle. While this taste-principle remains undissolved or strong, separated and uncompounded, fevers are not healed.

> Those attacked by pungent and acrid acids suffer greatly from frenzy, from gnawings of the bowels and chest and from restlessness. No relief...until the acidity is purged away or calmed down and mixed with the other humours.[50]

Thus the author seems to consider tastes both in terms of their effects on the body and as indicators of unblended humours or secretions/fluids.

He also argues against medicine based on heat and cold because his experience tells him that hot things can have different tastes and effects, some insipid, some astringent, some causing flatulence. In other words, hot things do not all have the same

48. Ibid., 41.
49. Ibid., 45-47.
50. Ibid., 51.

powers or effects, or possibly several different tastes can have a heating effect. He prefers medicine based on qualities, particularly as tastes, these being a more reliable guide to effect. In chapter XVII he states

> the truth being that one and the same thing is both bitter and hot, or acid and hot, or salt and hot, with numerous other combinations and cold again combines with other powers. It is these that cause the harm.[51]

It is tempting here to wonder if this is a similar approach to the understanding of drugs based on tastes that we find in Ayurvedic medicine. As will be discussed below, there we find that each drug is known by one predominant taste and each taste has a specific effect on the body. The bitter taste is strongly cooling and drying, the pungent taste heating and drying, the sweet taste is mildly cooling and strongly nutritive, etc. However, it seems that apart from saying that cheese, or wine or whatever are not bad in themselves but only may be for certain individuals depending on their constitution (chapter XX), he does not relate tastes to specific foods and their qualities. However, he does state that the physician must know "what a man is in relation to foods and drinks and to habits generally, and what will be the effects of each on each individual." The author ends his treatise by saying that when a humour that is sweet naturally changes its form, it becomes not salt or astringent, but acid. Therefore, when a sweet remedy is the least suitable for treating, acid will be the next least suitable. The implication is that for treating certain conditions, the astringent will be the most suitable, being the taste farthest from the sweet. These statements suggest strongly that such detailed knowledge of taste effects was at least beginning to be developed and was part of the physician's professional repertoire.

There is another reference to sweet in *Airs, Waters, Places* (VIII):

> the lightest part of it [of the cloud moisture] remains, and is sweetened as the heat of the sun produces coction, just as all other things always become sweeter through coction.[52]

---

51. Ibid., 45-47.
52. Ibid., 93.

Sweet here is a positive quality indicating mildness, blending and balance. We find a similar idea of the corrective power of coction in such works as the *Epidemics* and others, which discuss the signs to be looked for in order to understand the progress of a disease. The pathological humours which emerge from the body's various eliminative channels, i.e. the fluids or substances in sputum, urine, faeces, are monitored to discover whether they are 'acrid' and unconcocted or concocted and sweet. This finds parallels in *Ancient Medicine* as will be discussed below.

Returning to *Ancient Medicine*, we note that there seems also to be confusion (or perhaps conflation) between the idea of humour and that of taste and effect in the body. As in *Epidemics*, the humours themselves are said to be acid, acrid, bitter or sweet in *Ancient Medicine*, and when uncompounded, unblended they become harmful. In chapter XIX, the writer states,

> as long as these bitter particles are undissolved, undigested and uncompounded, by no possible means can the pains and fevers be stayed. And those who are attacked by pungent and acrid acids suffer greatly from frenzy, from gnawing of the bowels and chest and from restlessness. No relief from these symptoms is secured until the acidity is purged away, or calmed down and mixed with the other humours.[53]

One wonders if the phyicians actually tasted some of the expelled humours as part of their observations, or if they relied on the testimony of the patient for this information. Unfortunately, the information here on taste and effects is suggestive only, being so bare. This work offers only a slight possibility that for some physicians, therapy was based on the tastes of deranged humours and the tastes of foods, drinks and drugs which were used to counteract them.

In other treatises we do find extra details of the specific tastes and the corresponding qualities, effects, powers of foods and drinks. *Regimen in Acute Diseases*, classifies wines according to whether they are sweet or vinous (sour like vinegar).

53. Ibid., 51.

Each has its different effects.

> Sweet wine causes less heaviness in the head than the vinous, goes to the brain less, evacuates the bowels more than the other, but causes swelling of the spleen and liver. It is not suited either to the bilious....

And 'astringent' dark wine may be used if

> there be no heaviness to the head, if the brain be not effected, nor the sputum checked, nor urine stopped, and if stools be rather loose,

In other words, if there is no stagnation in any of the eliminative channels. The drink oxymel, made of honey and vinegar and given in acute conditions, is distinguished between less and 'very acid', which causes sputum to come up and out, promoting lubrication. *Regimen in Acute Diseases* notes that the acidity of vinegar benefits 'bitter bile' more than 'black' (LXI).[54]

The author of *Regimen II* seems to agree, saying, in chapter LII:

> Acid wines cool, moisten and attenuate. They cool and attenuate by emptying the body of its moisture, they moisten from the water that enters with the wine....[whereas] Vinegar ...is binding rather than laxative because it affords no nourishment and is sharp [sour?].[55]

Generally he prefers to describe foods according to the moist-dry, heating-cooling, binding-loosening polarities, but occasionally he extends the use of tastes to foods and herbs:

> LIV: Wild vegetables that are sweet and also 'warming in the mouth' warm the body, where as those that have a "moist, cold and sluggish nature or strong smell, pass more easily by stool than by urine...those that are sharp and of a sweet smell [and presumably taste] pass easily by urine; those that are sharp [pungent] and dry in the mouth [astringent] are drying to the body; those that are acid [sour] are cooling."[56]

---

54. Jones (1981) vol. II 105, 107, 117. In the twentieth century, a similar drink enjoyed a renaissance after the publications of Dr. Jarvis' book, *Folk Remedies of Vermont,* in which he recommended cider vinegar and honey for a number of ailments.
55. Jones (1979) vol. IV 327.
56. Jones (1979) vol. IV 333.

> LV: the sharp [pungent] taste of radish melts phlegm; anise and coriander are hot and astringent; things sweet and warming pass easily by stool; things sharp and dry, or acid are cooling.[57]

> LV: things sweet, sharp, salt, bitter or harsh are said to be naturally heating whether they are dry or moist, while things acid, sharp, harsh, astringent open up and cleanse congestions.[58]

Here 'hot' probably means the pungent-hot taste, as does 'sharp'. However, the meaning of astringent is less clear since it can mean both a dry or sour taste on the tongue and a drying and gathering effect on body tissues. For example, in chapter XLV we find beans described as astringent because they produce only a small residue after digestion. Thus when basil is described as dry, hot and astringent it may mean that it has a drying effect, is pungent to taste and therefore warming, and also causes fewer residues after digestion (see discussion of *perissomata* below).

In *Affections*, 55 the actions of three specific tastes of foods are mentioned. Sour foods dry, contract and constipate; sharp ones thin the body by irritation, salty ones are laxative and diuretic.[59]

In practice, with the above knowledge, if, for example, a patient was having trouble passing urine, the physician would know not to give him moist, cold vegetables, but hot ones, possibly cooked with hot/pungent herbs. There is at least the suggestion here of treatment being based on the effects known tastes have in the body—a therapy based on the correspondence of various tastes of foods, drinks and herbs with their action in the body.

The author of *Nature of Man* lends support to this suggestion when he writes in chapter VI:

> For just as things that are sown and grow in the earth, when they enter it, draw each constituent of the earth which is nearest akin to it—these are the acid, the bitter, the sweet, the salt and so on—first the plant

57. Ibid., 329-331.
58. Ibid., 341.
59. Potter (1988) vol. V 83-84.

> draws to itself mostly that element which is most akin to it, and then it draws the other constituents also. Such too is the action of drugs in the body. Those that withdraw bile first evacuate absolutely pure bile, then bile that is mixed. Those that withdraw phlegm first withdraw absolutely pure phlegm and then phlegm that is mixed.[60]

This statement, in the book of the *Corpus* which elaborates most fully a firm scheme of four bodily humours, shows firstly that different plants are recognized by their strongest tastes, and further that it was also believed they contained the other tastes in them to lesser degrees. Secondly, it shows that treatment was based on knowing which drugs, i.e. plant medicines, would be able to draw which pure (isolated) therefore deranged humours out of the body: acid tasting plants would draw acid humours.

Although this model of food/drug-taste-effect may seem at first ridiculous from the point of view of modern medical knowledge, in terms of herbal medicine, it finds a place. It was probably based on empirical experience with foods and their effects and possibly suggests the basis on which the physicians developed their paradigm of qualities and effects. Riddle (1985) has suggested that the organisation of Dioscorides' herbal was based not on botany but on well-known physiological effects.[61] It may be that these effects were first intuited by taste. For example, as Riddle points out, the bitter taste of wild lettuce produces a cooling, though not astringent, effect. This correlates with the effect of the bitter taste on bile cited in *Nature of Man*: in the body the drug withdraws first the constitutent of the body most like itself, the bitter taste is used to cleanse the excess of bile, which is associated with fevers. The bitter tasting herb is used to cool fevers by cleansing the bile humour. Many mildly warming herbs such as anise, cinnamon, fennel are also sweet and such herbs are used to reduce excess phlegm. Unfortunately, in Dioscorides, tastes are not mentioned for every herb nor can they always be so clearly related to effects. Even so, in practice

60. Jones (1979) vol. IV 17-18.
61. Riddle (1985) 22-23.

the matter is not always that simple, there are exceptions to the rules. But tastes may have been the starting point. As we shall see Ayurvedic medicine encountered the same situation and found a special way of explaining the discrepancies it discovered. For the Greeks too, even irregularities in nature were part of nature's rational order.[62]

In summary, while tantalising, the mention of different tastes in the Hippocratic writings does not seem to amount to the thoroughly worked-out scheme of tastes related to actions that we find in Āyurveda, although the statement from *Nature of Man* reveals that there may have been some development towards this. In one sense, however, the two schools of medicine do agree that tastes and their effects are more complicated than at first meets the eye.

## Pathological Digestion by Surfeit

The author of *Regimen III* claims to have made the discovery of

> how to diagnose what is the overpowering element in the body, whether exercises overpower food or food overpowers exercises; how to cure each excess and to insure good health so as to prevent the approach of disease, unless very serious and many blunders be made.[63]

Excess initiates disease by impairing proper coction. If food overpowers exercise, the disturbance can lead to a surfeit which 'gathers together', and which the body then expels as secretions.[64] In other words an excess is created which produces stagnation, in one case of the respiratory passages (mucus and saliva),[65] in another excessive sleep which while at first pleasant, eventually 'disturbs the soul' and thus sleep and the man is 'near an illness', the nature of which "depends on the secretion and the part that it overpowers."[66] We find a similar outlook in

62. Lloyd (1991) 424.
63. Jones (1979) vol. IV 367.
64. Ibid., 384 *plesmone* and *sullegomene.*
65. Ibid., 385.
66. Ibid., 389.

*Affections*, 47 which states: "Whichever food the cavity masters (i.e., digests fully), the body accepts (assimilates), producing not flatulence or colic."[67]

Surfeit (excess) sometimes brings on aches either in parts or all over the body, accompanied by fatigue. If a person feels fatigued, but instead of abstaining from eating, 'adopts a treatment of rest and over feeding', they 'fall into a fever', and "indulging in baths and food they turn the illness into pneumonia".[68] The patient here is clearly seen to be responsible for his condition and this recalls the words of *Regimen in Health* that "a wise man should consider that health is the greatest of human blessings, and learn how by his own thought to derive benefit in his illnesses". The author goes on to describe ten other 'types of surfeit' and their treatment with special foods according to taste and quantity, and treatment with vomiting, purges, massages and appropriate exercise.

The author of *Nature of Man* also recognized that excess was a major cause of disease when he stated:

> one must know that diseases due to repletion are cured by evacuation and those due to evacuation are cured by repletion.... Diseases in some cases arise from regimen and in some cases from air by the inspiration of which we live... (IX).[69]

In *Ancient Medicine*, as we have seen, the danger from separation of any part from its proper blending with others is seen to lead to 'overpowering' by one element of the others, whether that element be food, the different constituents or tastes of food, exercise, or sleep. Any of these states can lead to disease through surfeit, most commonly, though sometimes depletion can be the result.

---

67. Potter (1988) 71.
68. Jones (1979) vol. IV 391.
69. Jones (1979) vol. IV 25. The term *diaitematon* here can also mean more generally lifestyle habits which include diet. But since above the author referred to disease caused by excess, or repletion, we understand it here to refer to food.

## PATHOLOGICAL DIGESTION

### Pathological Digestion by Melting

In a kind of pathological reverse process of proper digestion and formation of tissues, tissues once formed are said to be capable of 'melting' and forming fluid secretions, i.e., converting into harmful isolated or separated humours. This will be discussed more fully in Chapter Four on the humours. Again here the idea seems to be that the fluid thus created, being now unblended and de-concocted, causes harm.

### Pathological Digestion Producing Residues

The idea of thorough digestion and assimilation leading to health through the good nutrition of all tissues in the body via the blood had an important corollary. This was the experience that if digestion was faulty, whether by wrong proportion of exercise, or wrong foods, or foods wrongly cooked, the effect would be the creation of waste matter from improperly digested, unassimilated food. In a case described in *Regimen III*, LXXIV, this 'rejected' nutriment, first produces flatulence but could gradually collect to a surfeit which then generates heat and affects the whole body, causing diarrhoea.[70] Another source for fifth century medicine is the text *Anonymus Londinensis*. It records that Euryphon and later Herodicus attribute disease to either nutriments not discharged by the belly but left as residues (Euryphon), or nutriment not assimilated but remaining and turning to residues (Herodicus). Herodicus further believed that the residues produce two liquids, an acid and a bitter, which have different effects according to their strength, their blending and the different places where they occur or lodge, for example in the head, liver or spleen.[71] Euryphon felt it was important that "when the belly is empty and clean/*lepte kai kathara*,

70. Jones (1979) vol. IV 395, 397 *sapeisa*, waste matter.
71. Phillips (1973) 32-33, based on Menon's text *Anonymus Londinensis* IV, 31-40 (Jones 1947). An extremely interesting discussion of this topic is found in *The Modern Hippocratic Tradition* by Wesley Smith. He finds a correspondence between the Hippocrates of *Regimen* and both Plato (the *Timaeus*) and Menon. Based on this he argues that *Regimen* is written by Hippocrates.

digestion takes place as it should."[72] If the belly is empty, one wonders what was there to be digested. Perhaps he is referring to the continuing sequential digestion and poor nutrition of tissues.

Although we find little or no such explanation of formation of residues in the Hippocratic texts, the fact that the basis of much of the treatment is cleansing of the bowels and stomach by means of emetics and purging herbs or enemas indicates that the presence of impurities or imbalances in the digestive tract, considered due to poor food or digestion, was a major component of Hippocratic medicine. Such purging is certainly a marked feature of Hippocratic treatment methods. It is the usual method used in fevers to clear the pathological humours, waste matters or residues.

However, these must first become concocted and compounded before they are stimulated to move. To allow this, a therapeutic fast is initiated based on barley gruel, *ptisane* (see below p. 122). Sometimes the gruel regimen is interrupted in order to administer the purges presumably because some at least of the pathological humours are ready to be cleansed—and then resumed again.[73] Sometimes, if food remains in the bowels, the gruel cannot be given until this food has first been purged; otherwise it will cause more pain.[74]

We find a similar idea in *Ancient Medicine*. The author may have had these ideas in mind when he spoke of acid, bitter, acrid humours produced by wrong diet. Such humour secretions may be in effect the equivalent of Herodicus' *perissomata*, i.e., the formation of pathological material in the digestive tract which needs to be removed or cleansed before proper digestion-assimilation can be restored.

## Pathological Digestion by Pneuma

In *Anonymus Londinensis*, chapters 5 and 6 credit another pathway by which food and digestion can imbalance the body, thus creating disease.

72. Menon IV 31-40 quoted in Smith (1973) 51.
73. Jones (1981) vol. II 71.
74. Ibid., 75.

5.35 But Hippocrates says that the cause of disease is gas (*phusa*), as Aristotle reports him. For Hippocrates says that diseases are brought about in the following fashion: either because of the quantity/*plethos* of things taken, or the diversity/*poikilia* or because they are strong and hard to digest, *perissomata* are produced.
5.44 And when the things taken are too many, the heat that effects digestion is overcome by so much food, and does not effect digestion. And because it is hindered, *perissomata* are produced.
6.4 And when the things taken are varied, they quarrel/*stasiazei* among themselves in the belly, and from the quarrel comes change into *perissomata*.
6.7 When foods taken are difficult to digest, there is hindrance of the digestion because of the difficulty of digestion, and thus a change into *perissomata*.
6.11 And from the *perissomata*, gas rises up, and the gas arising brings on diseases.[75]

Compare these reports of Hippocratic thinking with passages in *Regimen I* and *Breaths*.

*Regimen* (75, Littré, 6.616) There also occurs the following kind of *plesmone*: the next day food is belched up raw but not acid.... In this case the belly is cold and cannot digest food in the night. (56, Littré, 570) Meats in sauces cause burning and water, since fat, fiery and warm foods which have powers opposite to one another are residing together, (74. Littré, 614-616) There also occurs this kind of *plesmone*: when the food digests in the belly but the flesh does not receive it, the nourishment stays and makes gas *phusa*.[76]

These words are echoed in chapter 7 of the Hippocratic treatise *Breaths*. The author credits other dietary imbalances, which interfere with proper digestion and thus lead to disease.

75. Smith (1979) 52-53, Jones (1947) 35-37.
76. Ibid., 53, 54. Smith states that *Regimen* is the only work in the *Corpus* to express this theory of *perissomata* producing *phusa*.

> This is bad regimen, when one gives more wet or dry food to the body than it can bear, and opposes no labor to the quantity of nourishment. Also when one ingests foods that are varied/*poikilas* and dissimilar. Dissimilar things quarrel/*stasiazei* and some are digested faster, some slower...When the body is full of food it becomes full of *pneuma* when the foods remain too long...because its quantity keeps it from passing through. When the lower intestine is blocked air/*phusai* rushes through the whole body and falls on the parts that are full of blood and chills them.[77]

Ingestion of excess food means intake of excess air. The author of this work attributes the fundamental cause of all disease to derangements of air, an idea that we will examine more closely when we compare the Hippocratic and Ayurvedic concepts of humours in Chapter Four.

In this passage, what is most interesting for today's practitioner of complementary medicine is that the Hippocratic writers link the derangement of air to the digestive process, showing how its proper quantity and flow within the body can be imbalanced by poor eating habits and bad digestion. The point about foods of wide varieties eaten together is particularly interesting for two reasons. First, a very similar description of foods quarreling was given by an Ayurvedic lecturer; in this case he said that one reason foods are sometimes cooked together into soups or stews is that the foods settle their differences in the cooking pot, so when they are taken into the body, they are already at peace with one another.[78] Secondly, many symptoms of disease, such as skin and digestive problems, have been linked to food 'allergens'. Some people find that eating dairy or wheat/gluten products, for example, makes their problems much worse. Dr. William Howard Hay has based a diet on not eating starches and animal proteins in the same meal.[79] This has proved very effective in reducing or removing symptoms in many people. Others have focused on an imbalance of acid and alkaline-forming

77. Ibid., 53.
78. UK lecture by Dr. Robert Svoboda, December, 1993.
79. Grant and Joice (1991).

foods eaten together as a cause of or factor in certain diseases. Even epilepsy has been linked to nutritional deficiencies by one leading nutritionist. One reason behind the concept of fasting on a mono diet, prescribed by many practitioners, including medical doctors of 'ecological medicine', is that it allows the body to rest from having to digest so many foods. In this way the digestion is improved, fewer negative effects of digestion (*perissomata*) are produced to imbalance the body, and health restored. The Hippocratic prescription of barley gruel would also come into this category of a healing, mono diet. Thus the basic idea of the Hippocratic writers that not only good food (suited to the individual) but thorough digestion is necessary to keep the body healthy—and its corollary, disease may be treated via diet—can be seen to be viable and valid today.

## Food, Mind and Soul

One of the features of holistic medicine noted in the opening chapter was the taking into consideration of the mental-emotional state of the person when evaluating illness and diseased states, whether they be minor or major conditions. We have seen in Chapter One that the mental and spiritual sphere was an accepted part of the 'nature of man' which philosophers and physicians sought to understand. We now investigate if there is a similar awareness of and connection made between the mental-emotional and spiritual aspects of patients and their diet in health and disease.

If we first look for such ideas in the very treatises devoted to diet, we do indeed find that along with the ideas about purely physical causes of health and disease and the treatments, there is reference made to the other aspects of man's nature. Indeed *Regimen I,* II states:

> I maintain that he who aspires to treat correctly of human regimen must first acquire knowledge and discernment of the nature of man in general-knowledge of its primary constituents and discernment of the components by which it is controlled for if he is ignorant of primary constitution, he will be unable to gain knowledge of their effects and if

> he be ignorant of the controlling things in the body he will not be capable of administering to the patient suitable treatment.[80]

This treatise contains a marked philosophic element.[81] In Chapter VI, it is stated:

> All things are set in due order both the soul of man and likewise his body. Into man enter the parts of parts and the wholes of wholes.

In chapter VII the author writes, "Into man there exists a soul having fire and water." Chapter XXVIII continues, "soul is the same in all living creatures, although the body of each is different." Even blending affects the soul: "Blending affects the soul's intelligence, regimen makes the blending better or worse" (XXXVI). And in XXXV:

> The facts are as follows with regard to what are called the intelligence of the soul and the want of it. The moist fire and the driest water, when blended in a body, result in the most intelligence, because the fire has the moisture from the water and the water the dryness from the fire...The soul blended of these is most intelligent and has the best memory.[82]

Other treatises also show a knowledge of and interest in the relationship between diet and mental-spiritual states. In *Regimen III*, we find bodily states can affect the soul. Considering the negative effects of surfeit of food over exercise, the author states:

> when the body can no longer contain the surfeit, it now gives a secretion inwards through the force of the circulation, which, being opposed to the nourishment from food, disturbs the soul.... for as the experiences of the body are so are the visions of the soul when sight is cut off (LXXI).[83]

---

80. Jones (1979) vol.IV 227
81. Ibid., xxiv
82. Ibid., 239, 241, 267, 293, 281-283 respectively. Jones explains in his footnote, p. 281, that *phronesis* seems to mean the power of the soul to perceive things, whether by the mind or by the senses. He is unhappy with his translation. p. 20 "we lack terms like *phronein* for the complex unity which is the reality." Here perhaps we have the Greeks thinking more holistically.
83. Ibid., 389.

In *Humours* we find that unwise choices of food are attributed to 'psychical symptoms', i.e., if a physician observes such symptoms, he may conclude that there is an imbalance in the body: "Among psychical symptoms are intemperance in drink and food, in sleep, in wakefulness...." Furthermore, emotions specifically affect the body: "Accidents grieving the mind, fears, pains, pleasures, etc. to each of these the body responds by its *actions* [emphasis mine]". The author further notes, chapter XV, that "it is changes that are chiefly responsible for diseases, especially the greatest changes, the violent alterations both in the seasons and in other things" (for example, emotions or diet as above p. 55).[84] In *Affections* chapter 46 we read that both food and drink are to be administered to the patient in accordance with their body and their spirit "for in this way they are helped most."[85]

The author of *Breaths* discusses epilepsy, a disease affecting consciousness most dramatically, as based ultimately on deranged air, which in turn affects phlegm in the brain. For this author, as discussed above (p. 56) consciousness is intimately connected to breath and air, and can be deranged by poor food combinations, and quantities affecting digestion and the intake and distribution of air.

*Regimen IV* is especially interesting from the point of view of mind–body connection for it explicitly bases health assessment on mental–emotional states as revealed in dreams (LXXXVI). These can be directly related to foods. If things that appear in dreams are pure, then that shows that what has entered into, or happens to the body is also pure and healthful:

> Whatsoever a man seems to receive pure from a pure god is good for health; for it indicates that the matter is pure that enters the body (LXXXIX).[86]

Equally, imbalances in the body can be assessed by understanding dreams, for what is imbalanced in the body will affect the soul. In chapter LXXXVIII he writes that certain dreams indicate

84. Ibid., 81,89.
85. Potter (1988) vol.V 71, spirit/*psuche*.
86. Jones (1979) vol. IV 435.

> a disturbance in the body.... For a disturbance of the soul has been caused by a secretion arising from some surfeit that has occurred.[87]

Treatment is a cleansing emetic, then a light diet and exercise regime, gradually increased to vigorous, and finally voice exercises. This last suggests an awareness of the connection between breath–soul–consciousness and vocal expression. This author exemplifies the mixture of reverence for the divine in life with the practicalities of taking responsibility for one's health when he says, "Prayer is indeed good but while calling on the gods, a man should himself lend a hand."[88]

The author of *Epidemics* 2, 6.5 also relates in more general terms good sleep with health when he uses the metaphor of food nourishment: "Labour is food for the joints and the flesh, sleep for the intestines."[89]

## Stress or Trauma and Diet

Both *Regimen in Health* and *Regimen in Acute Diseases* would agree with the author of *Humours*, for each emphasised that imbalances, and thus disease, can be caused by any sudden change from what is habitual, in this case the habits of foods consumed and number of meals taken in a day. Diarrhoea, for example, can be caused because "digestive organs have been loaded, contrary to habit, when they are accustomed to a period of dryness and not to be twice distended with food and to digest food twice."[90] *Regimen in Health* seeks to offset the shock to the system that changes of seasons necessarily bring by moderating the diet. The author of *Aphorisms* would concur, for Chapter LI, Book II states:

> excess and suddenness in evacuating the body or in replenishing, warming or cooling or in any other way disturbing it is dangerous, in fact all excess is hostile to nature. But 'little by little' is a safe rule, especially in cases of change from one thing to another.[91]

---

87. Ibid., 425.
88. Ibid., 423.
89. Smith (1994) 257.
90. Jones (1981) vol. II 87. See also p. 91: "The chief causes of disease are the most violent changes in what concerns our constitutions and habits."
91. Jones (1979) 121.

This 'any other way'. could presumably include excessive emotions. Strong emotions, for example were thought by Greek writers to affect the liver/bile and the lungs, and physicians sometimes treated the patient through the emotions.[92] This attitude to change perhaps represents the acute awareness on the part of these ancient physicians of the subtle but significant effects that stress or trauma, whether emotional, dietary or seasonal, can have on the body—enough to result in a diseased condition.

From the above excerpts we can see that the Hippocratic physician felt he needed to know what his patients 'were' by what they were eating. He also perceived both that their minds affected their food and diet, and that their foods affected their mental–emotional states, and even their very soul. The physician would devise his prescriptions of food and drink, bearing in mind the mental state of his patient and the effect the substances would have upon it.

## Theory in Practice: Barley Gruel Treatment for Fevers

Before we leave this topic of food and health, let us finally consider in more detail a characteristic therapeutic approach of the *Corpus* and see if it can be better understood in the light of the foregoing.

The fasting treatment we find throughout the *Corpus*, Jones has called 'starvation'—an unhappy translation since the effect is to belittle the treatment. He also wrote that "to prevent auto-intoxication from undigested food—this was about all ancient medicine could accomplish, at least on the material side."[93] Yet basing a therapy on cleansing the digestive tract, by means of both fasting and herbs, to restore its proper environment is a major component of Ayurvedic medicine. It has also long been a treatment in naturopathic medicine. The relationship between disorder in the digestive tract and illness is increasingly accepted even by conventional medicine today.

Evidently the physician did not see such treatment as starvation, nor as 'about all' he could do, but as a most effective means

---

92. Onians (1994) chapters V, III and *Epidemics* 2.4.4. Smith (1994) 73.
93. Jones (1981) xiii.

of dealing with conditions caused by surfeit and also for acute, life-threatening fevers. The treatment did not, in fact, consist of 'starvation' but rather of a prescribed fast based on feeding the patient a mono-diet of a very special food, barley gruel or *ptisane*. This food was chosen for its specific qualities and virtues which made it the ideal food for such conditions.

Barley gruel is the main topic of discussion in *Regimen in Acute Diseases* between chapters VI and XXVII. The author states his reasons in chapter X:

> Now I think that gruel/*ptisane* made from barley has rightly been preferred over other cereal foods in acute diseases...for the gluten of it is smooth, consistent, soothing, lubricant, moderately soft, thirst-quenching, easy of evacuation, should this property too be valuable and it neither has astringency [as in the astringency of beans, *Regimen II*, XLV] nor causes disturbance in the bowels or swells up in them.[94]

In chapter XV, he adds: "In addition to its excellent lubricating qualities the best boiled gruel quenches thirst the most, is the most easily digested, and the least disturbing. All these characteristics are needed."[95]

In acute fevers, patients would then consume this gruel, usually without intermission, unless it was necessary to administer other treatments, such as cleansing the bowels with herbs or enemas (XI), until there were signs of improvement and the *krisis* occurred. The crisis was a positive event that signified that the humours had become concocted and any element in isolation had become re-compounded and blended. They would then be able to move towards the elimination channels where they could be helped to leave the body by the physician, again using herbs to induce a cleansing vomiting and/or purging of the bowels (XI). Signs of improvement include a moist mouth and sputum (the more liquid the sputum, the more easily it is eliminated). Early abundant moisture indicates an early crisis, in which case,

94. Jones (1981) vol. II 71.
95. Jones (1981) vol. II 75.

the instructions are to increase the quantity of gruel. When purging of bowels is administered, the gruel should be fed again afterwards (to renourish the body), and if the purging is complete, the quantity gruel is duly increased (XII). In this way the physician prevented the patient from excess elimination, which would only deplete the body.

Very detailed information is given on how to prepare the gruel and whether to give it as 'pure juice', i.e., strained barley water, or unstrained. When to give it is also carefully explained. Wrong administration can be dangerous (XVII). The right time for administering the gruel must be carefully observed from the beginning of the illness and throughout its course (XX). It is important not to give the gruel unless the bowels be empty of food (XIX). It should not be given if the feet are cold (elsewhere coldness of extremities is a sign of death, and since barley is cold, it would only worsen this). It should be given when the heat of the fever descends to the feet (XX). The protocols are given: best practice is to begin administering the gruel at the beginning of the disease rather than after fasting for two or three days, as some physicians do. By following this procedure, the change is brought about correctly and surely (XXVII). One is reminded of the admonition to proceed little by little in *Aphorisms* II, 2. Here the idea of change could be referring to the crisis of the fever, though the word *krisis* is not used.

In the works *Epidemics* I and III-which record many cases of fevers, probably malarial—we have descriptions of the general types and characters of diseases in specific places (the 'constitutions' of the disease and the locality), as well as detailed observances of the progress of individual cases. Surprisingly, very little mention is made of treatment, but as Jones says,

> we must not suppose that the fatally stricken patients of the *Epidemics* received no treatment or nursing. Here and there the treatment is mentioned or hinted at, but the writer assumes that the usual methods were followed and does not mention them because they are irrelevant.[96]

96. Jones (1971) vol. I xviii-xix.

However in books of the *Corpus* such as *Aphorisms, Diseases III*, and *Internal Affections* details of treatment for various conditions including fevers are given. Parts of *Diseases III* are considered to be physician's handbooks.[97] In it, for treating pneumonia, the following instructions are given:

> Begin by lightening the head in order that no flux to the chest will occur. On the first days, gruels should be sweetish, for with these you will best wash away and remove what has been deposited and congealed in the chest; on the fourth and fifth, change from sweet to rich ones, for this helps the patient to cough up sputum gently; if he is unable to expectorate as he should give expectorant medications. In the first four or five days, you must evacuate the cavities and quite well, in order that the fevers will be blunted and the pains lightened. However, when the body has been emptied and is weak, move the lower cavity down gently only every other day, in order that the body will retain some strength and that the upper regions will remain adequately moist.... In short the lower cavity can neither be allowed to remain inactive—to prevent the fevers from being too sharp, nor be too thoroughly evacuated—in order that the sputum will be able to be expectorated and the patient will remain strong.[98]

In *Aphorisms* we find more detail on how fasting or 'restricted regime' was employed and the attention to the minutest nuance is impressive. Section I.VI states that "for extreme diseases extreme strictness of treatment is most efficacious". I.VII goes on

> where disease is very acute, immediately, ...it is essential to employ a regimen of extreme strictness...when the disease is at its height that it is necessary to use the most restricted regimen.

But I.IX cautions: "Take the patient too into account and decide whether he will stand the regimen at the height of the disease".

---

97. Potter (1988) vol. VI 4.
98. Ibid., 35, 37.

The regimen implemented was varied as the disease progressed or changed its nature: I.XI states, "lower diet during exacerbation, for to give food is harmful...."[99]

Such treatments were not applied arbitrarily or haphazardly, but with due regard to the nature of the disease and of the individual patient (age, constitution). For example, I.XIII reminds the physician that old men endure fasting most easily, while those of middle age and the young very badly; children bear it worst of all. I.III similarly cautions that 'reduction of flesh' to extremes is treacherous; it need only be to a point compatible with the constitution of the patient. Section II.IV states the fundamental principle: "Neither repletion, nor fasting, nor anything else is good when it is "too great for the constitution or more than natural."[100]

The diet recommended by the author for fevers is "a sloppy or moist diet" (I.XVI) – in other words, probably the barley *ptisane*, or foods made moist by certain cooking preparations, though some food can be given according "to season, district, habit and age" (I.XVII). The physicians also knew to lessen carefully the diet before a crisis (I.XIX). In VII.LXVI, we have what may be the source of the expression 'starve fever, feed a cold' for the author states:

> If you give a fever patient the same food as you would to a healthy person, it is strength to the healthy but disease to the sick.[101]

Here we have an important concept in traditional medicine, found also in Indian medicine: do not give food or medicine which adds to the strength of the disease.

If we compare these instructions with those for acute fevers in, for example, *Regimen in Acute Diseases* we can see that they are broadly similar, being based on giving gruel and cleansing the bowels and regulating treatment according to the constitution, habits and age of the patient, the season, and the progress of the disease (i.e., near the crisis). Most modern scholars examining

---

99. Jones (1979) vol. IV 103-105.
100. Ibid., 105, 103, 109.
101. Ibid., 107, 211.

the *Corpus* consider that the Hippocratic physician was practising the best medicine he could under the circumstances. That is, knowledge of germ pathology was lacking, and the physician had no other choice but to "hinder Nature as little as possible in her efforts to expel a disease...."[102] However, as Phillips has pointed out, before the advent of antibiotics within the last fifty years, similar methods of treatment were still being employed "within living memory".[103] In spite of the advances in treating acute conditions with antibiotic medicine, some natural medicine practitioners have continued this tradition, even if they have had to be on the fringes of society. Again in certain diseases, such as Crohn's, while some hospitals treat with a drug therapy, others, notably Addenbrooke's in Cambridge, have adopted an approach which includes management of diet.[104] Recently, aggressive antibiotic therapy has been shown to have its limitations: (not only have bacteria quickly developed resistance, but the antibiotics wipe out the friendly bacteria in the body which would be working to overcome the infection, leaving the patient completely exposed).[105]

Having established the protocols of Hippocratic treatment and the reasons behind them, we may now look into the sources of Ayurvedic tradition to discover if there exist similar ideas and treatment methods.

---

102. Jones (1981) vol. II, xiii.
103. Phillips (1973) 84. Such practices are preferred by many naturopaths, herbalists and homeopaths today.
104. Craik (1995, Powell) 397-401 has also pointed out certain correspondence between contemporary medical and nutritional knowledge about diet and those in the Hippocratic corpus.
105. For example, the case of a person with bactérial infection secondary to hospitalisation for mild heart attack was admitted to a hospital in Scotland from Spain. Antibiotics failed to kill the infection and three other patients in the intensive care ward with the new patient were infected. The heart attack victim and two of the patients died. The consultant only managed to save the life of the last patient by stopping the use of all antibiotics—contrary to protocol—thus allowing the victim's own bacteria and immune system to overcome the pathogenic bacteria. Reported on "You and Yours", Radio 4, 30 May, 1996.

## AYURVEDIC CONCEPTS ABOUT FOOD, NUTRITION AND DISEASE IN *'CARAKA SAṂHITĀ'*

That the foundation of health and a fundamental cause of disease is food, wholesome or unwholesome, is attested many times in *Caraka*. Several chapters are devoted to food, diet, seasonal factors, and so on. Sūtrasthāna, chapter XXVII, verses 349-350 states: "food sustains the life of living beings. Complexion, clarity, good voice, longevity, geniusness, happiness, satisfaction, nourishment, strength and intellect are all conditioned by food."[106] Chapter XXVIII, verses 45-48, states:

> The body as well as diseases are caused by food; wholesome and unwholesome foods are responsible for happiness and misery respectively.[107]

The author, in chapter XXVII, lists various foods, drinks, dairy products, fruits, etc. and their effects on the body in terms of their *vīrya, doṣa,* actions and qualities among the the twenty pairs of opposites derived from the five great elements. For the proper nutrition of the body, and for individual types of bodies (constitutions/*prakṛti*) we find in the texts foods classified according to their qualities of hot-cold, moist-dry and according to tastes. For example, in Sūtrasthāna I, chapter XXV, verses 35-37, we find a list of twenty food items, among them rice, pulses, salts, meats, fats and oils, vegetables, sugars and fruits. Another list presents one hundred and fifty-six herbs as well as foods and their effects. The effects include emotional states such as grief and happiness.[108]

Earlier in the chapter, foods are said to have six tastes, and twenty qualities.[109] The competent physicians will know the food

106. Sharma and Dash (1995) vol. I 565.
107. Ibid., 583.
108. Ibid., 423-435. The list enumerates a wide variety of items according to whether and how they benefit health. Other items include roots, barks, habitual use of milk, ghee, meat; massage, feelings such as grief, worry, baths, enemas, fevers, types of geography.
109. Ibid., 422. The six tastes are: sweet, astringent, salty, pungent, bitter and sour. The qualities are the standard twenty of the cosmos in general: heaviness/lightness, cold/hot, unctuousness/dryness, dullness/sharpness, stability/fluidity, softness/hardness, subtlety/grossness, solidity/liquidity, non sliminess/sliminess, roughness/smoothness.

articles, their properties, action, dosage in all respects (verse 35). Food articles which maintain the equilibrium of bodily *dhātus* and "help in eliminating the disturbance of their equilibrium" are the wholesome ones (verses 33-34). Here we find the concept of balance among various factors as being most essential to good health. The list of food qualities is similar to, but more extensive than, that of the Hippocratic treatises. Numerology was important to Hippocratic writers but mainly in respect to critical days or periods of time in a disease, or in ideas of embryology. In Āyurveda, numerology is taken to much greater lengths and this is reflected in the enumeration of twenty qualities of foods. In fact these remind us of the twenty qualities of substances we find in the descriptions of the nature of the *kosmos* according to Presocratic thinkers.

The Hippocratic model of a process of bodily nourishment via the transformative action of digestive fire, i.e., cooking, first in the stomach but also in subsequent other bodily tissues, bears a remarkable resemblance to the description of "*dhātu* nutrition" found in the Ayurvedic classic text, *Caraka Saṃhitā*. *Dhātu* means tissue and there are seven in the body: *rasa/ chyle-juice, rakta*/blood, *māṃsa*/muscle, *medas*/fats, *asthi*/bone, *majjan*/ marrow, *śukra*/semen. Breastmilk is considered a *upadhātu* or secondary tissue of *rasa*.

## Tissue Nutrition

The digestive process has been likened by one contemporary teacher of Āyurveda to the processing of milk in different ways and stages to produce different products, i.e., raw milk makes yoghurt, yoghurt is churned to make butter (in India), butter is cooked to make ghee, or clarified butter. (Ghee is considered to be a superior medicinal product and is the vehicle for many other medicinal preparations.) In this process the idea is that the essence of the material (initially the foodstuff, subsequently the *dhātu*), at each stage nourishes or forms the next tissue.[110]

*Agni* is the term for digestive fire, or enzymes of digestion (named after or internalised from of the fire god, Agni). In Āyurveda, not only the stomach has *agni*, but each tissue element has its own element of *agni* so that it may engage in a further digestive

110. Sharma and Dash (1995) vol. I 568, Sūtrasthāna XXVIII, 4.

process through which it is nourished by the previous tissue, and provides nourishment for the successive tissue. The formation of these tissues is seen as a progressive cycle of digestion. Thus *agni* in the stomach transforms food into *rasa* (chyle). *Rasa agni* transforms a bit of *rasa* into *rakta* or blood. *Rakta agni* transforms a bit of *rakta* into muscle. *Māṃsa agni* transforms a bit of itself into fats, and so on. At each stage, waste products are formed and a more refined or 'purified' portion forms the next tissue until finally the last tissue *śukra* is transformed into *ojas* or vital fluid essence, the most refined and dynamic substance of the body. (Today it is related to the body's immune strength and overall vitality, often as reflected in sexual potency.) There are various channels of circulation, or *srotas*, and the nutriment is carried to the *dhātu* by and through these channels.[111]

This concept of a progression of subsequent digestions to form each bodily tissue is remarkably similar to that we find in the *Corpus* as previously discussed. By comparison it is more thoroughly and explicitly worked out in Āyurveda but this may be misleading. We must remind ourselves that in *Caraka* we have a compendium of differing views and traditions which have already been to some extent melded, whereas in the *Corpus*, the independently written treatises preserve their individuality and reveal the differences among the physicians.

## Aetiology of Disease from Pathological Digestion

An image used by a contemporary teacher of Āyurveda, when discussing digestion and transformation of food into tissue, is that of a fire with a cooking pot of rice.[112] For example, if any aspect of the process is imperfect, i.e., the food in the pot is unwholesome for the individual, or other factors such as time of year, or state of mind are unfavourable, or there is too much or not enough food in proportion to water or the fire is either too hot or not hot enough, the food in the pot will not be properly cooked. The same is said to happen in the 'cooking pot' of the

111. Ibid. 568-573, Sūtrasthāna XXVIII, 4-5.
112. Lectures of Dr. Vasant Lad, Sept. 1992.

body, the stomach through the 'power of digestion'.[113] If at any stage in this process digestion and *dhātu* formation is not complete, due to "low *agni*" or other factors, then several different consequences are described in different parts of the text. One of these is that the channels through which nutrition for the *dhātus* is to flow can become blocked, and this can lead to diseased states.[114] Another is that the *doṣa,* or humours of *vāta, pitta, kapha*/air, fire, water become vitiated and cause imbalance.[115] Another is that *ama* is formed. Since *ama* seems to bear a resemblance to our Greek concept *perissomata,* we will consider it in more detail.

'*Ama*' means raw or incompletely processed residues of digestion, and when present, *ama* becomes a cause of disease, because it stagnates and clogs the channels by its congestion. One of the words used for disease is *amaya* or that which is born out of *ama.* Causes of *ama* include undigested food, improper elimination, humour imbalance and repressed emotions.[116] According to Sūtrasthāna XIX, which lists numerous forms of disease such as fevers, abdominal, and urinary disorders, there are two types of diseases caused by *ama* or improper digestion and metabolism: *alasaka* (intestinal torpor) and *visūcikā* (choleric diarrhoea). In Vimānasthāna II such *ama* can also have a poisonous effect on the body, creating the disease known as *āmaviṣa.* In *alasaka,* "if a weak individual, having low power of digestion and excessive *kapha* in his body, suppresses the urge for voiding flatus, urine and stool, and takes compact, heavy, un-unctuous, cold and dried food in excessive quantity, food and drinks [in the digestive tract] get affected with *vāta.* Simultaneously the passage gets obstructed by *kapha* due to excessive adhesiveness of the food product."[117] In Passage 13 the treatment is given: "[it] should be treated with emesis in the beginning by administering hot saline water. Thereafter fomentation and suppositories should be employed and the

113. Sharma and Dash (1995) vol. I 562-563; 339-341, Sūtrasthāna XXVII.
114. Ibid., 572-573, Sūtrasthāna XXVIII, 4, 5, 581 XXVIII 33.
115. Ibid., 574, Sūtrasthāna XXVIII, 7.
116. Ibid., vol. II 134-137, Vimānasthāna 7, 8, 9, 10-12.
117. Ibid., 136, 12.

patient should be made to fast."[118] In Cikitsāsthāna, III, 137-138 which is describing the signs and symptoms of *ama jvara* or the first stages of fever caused by *ama*, a sign that the patient has become free of *ama* are: "[re]appearance of appetite, lightness of the body, reduction in temperature, elimination of *doṣa* along with waste products from the body."[119]

This idea of *ama* as raw and therefore harmful seems therefore similar to the Greek idea of *perissomata*. Both traditions agree that the purpose of digestion is to 'cook' and transform foods into substances that can feed the body tissues; and that uncooked or poorly digested foods form harmful residues which can imbalance the body and initiate disease.

In Sūtrasthāna, verses XVIII 9-10 when the first *dhātu*, *rasa* (juice-chyle) gets vitiated, the disease that can result includes: disinclination for food, emaciation, nausea, heaviness, drowsiness, fever with malaise, obstruction of the *srotas* (channels of circulation), emaciation, loss of power of digestion. These are symptoms similar to those we find in the fever cases in the Hippocratic *Epidemics*. Thus unwholesome food and poor digestion producing an unwholesome residue is seen to be an important causative factor for fever.

## Food and the Treatment of Fevers

For treating fever, *jvara*, the classical text recommends first *langhana* or lightening therapy in the initial stages of the fever; in other words, fasting. (The exception is fevers with wasting signs, such as consumption.) This is because the stomach–small intestine is seen to be the site of origin of the disease. Such lightening diets were highly specific. In the opening chapter of the Nidānasthāna, or section of diagnosis, we find the discussion of fever. Under the heading of various types of exploratory therapy, *upaśaya*, for fever, the commentator expands the text by enumerating eighteen types of treatment in sets of three, drugs,

118. Ibid., 137, 138.
119. Ibid., vol. III, 148. The *doṣas* or humours being vitiated are also an important factor as they are in some Hippocratic treatises. They will be discussed in more detail in the chapter on humours.

diet and regimen (types of activities, e.g. sleeping or specific exercise). The diets are as follows: (1) diets antagonistic to the cause of disease: e.g., intake of meat soup in fever caused by fatigue and by vitiation of *vāta;* (2) diets antagonistic to the disease itself: e.g. intake of bowel-binding diets like *masūra* for diarrhoea; (3) diets antagonistic to both the disease and its cause: e.g. in fever caused by cold things intake of hot and antipyretic gruel; (4) diets which work against the causative factors of disease even though not actually antagonistic: e.g. intake of diets which cause heating sensation by a patient suffering from oedema.[120] This finely tuned dietary therapy was based on what the physician diagnosed as the cause or predisposing factor of the fever.

Treatment thereafter depends on the *doṣa* involved, but includes a choice of decoctions of herbs, drinks, unction, oleation therapy, fomentations, ointment, baths or application of pasted medicines, emesis, purgation, *āsthāpana* type of enema, alleviation therapy, inhalation, fumigation, smoking, collyrium, and milk preparations.[121]

One treatment is especially featured in the subsequent verses: *ghee*, or clarified butter. Ghee is said to be beneficial in all types of chronic fever but it has to be prepared by boiling with certain drugs to alleviate the particular *doṣa* involved. The reasons ghee is so useful are explained in detail in the accompanying commentary by Cakrapāṇidatta in which it is explained how the qualities of ghee, itself oily and warming (therefore normally aggravating to *pitta doṣa*), are rendered useful for each vitiated *doṣa* if prepared in the right way.[122]

Since there is no other feature of a single specific food used in the treatment of fevers, we may perhaps be permitted to assume that ghee holds a special place in treatment similar to that of barley gruel for the Hippocratic physician. Certainly today, ghee is held to be a useful cure all for all manner of conditions in India. However, gruels were also used therapeutically, including a gruel of barley. If we examine the chapters enumerating foods

120. Ibid., vol. II 9-10, Nidānasthāna I, 10-11.
121. Ibid., vol. II, 30-31, Nidānasthāna I, 36.
122. Ibid., vol. II 31-32, Nidānasthāna I, 37.

and their qualities, we do find that barley is said to be "unctuous, cold in potency, light and sweet accompanied with astringent taste. It produces wind and stool in large quantity. It is stabilising, and strength promoting."[123] It alleviates the vitiated *kapha doṣa*. *Kapha* is the *doṣa* (humour) that tends most to stagnation, and as such this may correspond to the state of surfeit of phlegm described by Hippocratic doctors, who also used barley similarly. The commentator, citing another roughly contemporaneous text, *Suśruta Saṃhitā* 46: 41, adds that barley is strength-promoting because it clarifies obstruction to the channels of circulation or because of its specific action. "[and]...it alleviates not only *kapha* but also pitta, curing adiposity, infections and toxic conditions."[124] In the chapter on preparation of alcohol-based medicines, we find a fermented barley gruel.[125] In chapter II, 17 of Sūtrasthāna we find an enumeration of different varieties of gruel and their use in disease. They are specifically to be used, the later commentator tells us, in cases of suppressed appetite and to alleviate colic pain.

> It has been said, 'as a small particle of fire is by and by kindled with the help of grass, cowdung, etc. so the inner fire, i.e., appetite, is enhanced and stabilised and is rendered all digestive with the help of medicated gruel in respect of a patient who has been purged [by the administration of elimination therapies].[126]

There follows a list of twenty-eight rice gruels prepared with various herbs, milk products, meat, oils, etc.[127] This is understandable, given that in India rice came to hold a place as dietary staple equivalent to that of barley in Greece. In a passage in Nidānasthāna on fever, we also find mention of the use of 'anti-pyretic gruel' along with herbs and diets antagonistic to the disease.[128] Chapter XXVII of Sūtrasthāna, verses 250-256 discusses the healthful properties of thin gruel: it

---

123. Ibid., vol. I, 496, Sūtrasthāna XXVII, 19, 20.
124. Ibid.
125. Ibid., 440 and 443, Sūtrasthāna XXV, 48, 49.
126. Ibid, 68.
127. Ibid. 69-70.
128. Ibid., vol. II, 10 (commentary to verse 10, no. 8).

> alleviates hunger, thirst-depression, weakness, abdominal diseases, and fever. It promotes sweating. It is digestive and is conducive to the downward movement of the flatus as well as faeces. Thick gruel is refreshing, bowel-binding, light and cardiotonic.[129]

Various gruels of rice specially prepared with different herbs are then described along with their effects.

Such detail in varieties and methods of preparation of medicinal gruel reveals that the physician required detailed knowledge to decide which to use, as well as when and how to administer it. This corresponds to what we found among Hippocratic physicians. We also find that there was a tradition of treating fevers through fasting on either rice or barley gruel in Āyurveda, comparable to that of Hippocratic medicine.

## Physician as Cook

As the above discussion also shows, the Ayurvedic physicians were of the same mind as the Hippocratic about the necessity for skill in preparing foods and medicines. At the end of Sūtrasthāna II we find:

> Only the physician endowed with memory, having adequate knowledge of causes of diseases and health and principles of propriety, self-restrained, and having presence of mind is entitled to practice medicine through the combination of various drugs.[130]

In chapter XXV, of Sūtrasthāna verses 26-29 of *Caraka* it states:

> the same factors, which, in the state of their *wholesome combination* are responsible for the creation of living beings, in the state of their *unwholesome combination* are responsible for the various diseases [emphasis mine][131]

Verse 36 enumerates the various ways foods may be defined, for example according to their tastes, qualities, the ways they are taken, or their habitats. The verse ends with the statement: "such

129. Ibid., 543.
130. Ibid., 73, Sūtrasthāna II, 36.
131. Ibid., 419.

variations are innumerable, depending upon the combination and preparation of food articles."[132] Since a large part of the information of diet therapy is concerned with describing how to combine and prepare foods to have certain effects, these skills of *saṃyoga*, combination and *karaṇa*, method of preparation, represent specialised knowledge of the skilled physician in Āyurveda much as they do for the Hippocratic.

## The Ayurvedic Concept of Tastes and Powers

One area where we do not find such extensive similarities between the two traditions is that of taste. As discussed above, there is a tantalising hint of a therapy based on taste in the treatise *Ancient Medicine*, and other books, such as *Regimen in Health*, do make reference to the taste of a food or drink in describing its therapeutic uses. Yet there is nothing comparable to the detailed model of the six tastes in Āyurvedic tradition. In *Caraka* each taste has a specific action in the body, so the effects of all foods, drinks, herbs can be known by their taste. This at first seems a tidy theory. However, experience has shown that things may not be this simple, since a notable concept is equally important in Āyurveda: the post-digestive effect of a taste-substance, its *vipāka*. This concept helps explain why the action of a substance does not always correspond to what would be expected according to its primary taste. The ancient physicians then were willing to adapt an explanation to take into account the practical realities they experienced. Thus certain substances are known to have certain effects regardless of their initial taste or *rasa*. In addition, actions of some substances experientially cannot be accounted for by even the *vipāka*, so another special factor is conceived—*prabhāva* or special potency. In effect the physician simply had to know the therapeutic effect of each drug based on practical experience of its action.

Such empirical knowledge may have been in the mind of the writer of *Ancient Medicine* when he decried the treatment method based on correspondence between heat and effects in the body, which was the approach of rival physicians. He notes that

---

132. Ibid., 422.

> one hot thing happens to be astringent, another hot thing insipid, and a third hot thing causes flatulence (for there are many various kinds of hot things, possessing many opposite powers)...for it is not the heat which possess the great power but the astringent and the insipid and the other qualities I have mentioned, whether eaten or drunk, whether applied externally as ointment or as plaster (Chapter XV).[133]

In this work the concept argued is one of 'powers' and these are defined in terms of tastes, although temperatures and even humours are also mentioned. We saw earlier examples in other treatises of how the physicians used tastes for their therapeutic effects. It could be said that the Greeks seem to put taste and *vipāka-prabhāva* together in their term *dunameis.*[134] At any rate there is a suggestion in this work of the beginnings of a model of therapy based on taste–*dunameis*, but it is not worked out with the detail which we find it in *Caraka*. The information in *Caraka* of the existence of a corresponding model of taste-effects, and their special exceptions, helps illuminate our understanding of what the Hippocratic physicians were aiming at and suggests it is more significant than would otherwise appear.

## A COMPARISON OF THERAPEUTIC REGIMENS FOR A CONDITION OF EXCESS

### Hippocratic

In *Regimen III*, for the overpowering of exercise by food the signs are the surfeit of phlegm and saliva: as the body is at rest, they block up the passages of the breath, the surfeit inside being considerable. For this congested condition—equivalent to our common cold—the author points out that exercise warms the humour (phlegm/mucus) so that it thins and separates itself out. Here we have in effect the cooking of the congested phlegm/mucus by the warmth/fire of exercise, which thins it out and prepares it for evacuation from the body. The treatment prescribed may be summarised as follows: exercise thoroughly, but

133. Jones (1972) vol. I 41.
134. I am indebted to Dr. J. M. Wilkins for this observation.

be careful to avoid fatigue; follow with a warm bath, then a varied meal and then emetic therapy. This is followed by a short walk in the sun. The next day take the same but lighter and less exercise and reduce dinner by one half.[135] From then daily food should be gradually increased.

This treatment may seem strange and even ineffectual to us today although perhaps not necessarily 'gentle'. However, if looked at in the light of Āyurveda, the treatment begins to make sense. Let us take it in its different aspects.

First, exercise is prescribed to warm the surfeit, thin it and cause it to be separated out. Actually, anyone with a slightly stuffy head who goes out and does exercise to get the blood moving will be able to testify to the effectiveness of this prescription in 'thinning' the mucous and separating it. An important precaution is that of avoiding fatigue.

Second, a warm bath is prescribed. Here too the therapeutic strategy is to keep the phlegm thin and separated. In addition the bath cleanses the skin, which was considered literally to 'breathe' through its pores and was hence a means of elimination.

Third, a varied meal is prescribed. It is not clear exactly what is meant by this, but the sense is of a meal of all sorts of foods.

Fourth, emesis or vomiting therapy is administered. This is the point that seems most strange.

Fifth, a light walk in the sun is prescribed. Again the aim is to keep the body and the humour mildly warm, yet relaxed, not over-exerting.

The fourth procedure seems most strange, but let us see what light Ayurveda can shed on the thinking behind it.

## Ayurvedic

In Āyurveda, the stomach is considered to be the site of the water–earth humour, *kapha*. *Kapha* is most recognisable in the body as mucus with its qualities of coldness, and moistness. The primary site of *kapha* in the body is the stomach, where digestion of food takes place.

Āyurveda recognises that each *doṣa*, e.g. *kapha*, is necessary

135. Most Greeks habitually ate only one or two meals a day.

in the body, but when it becomes disordered it causes problems. Evidently the connection between vitiated *kapha* and head complaints was well-known to the ancient writer of *Caraka* because in one passage, describing the treatment of kapha disease it is stated that treatment is by therapies "like fomentation, emesis, elimination of dosas from the head, exercise and so on".... The passage goes on to state that of

> all the devices stated above, emetic therapy is the treatment par excellence for the cure of diseases due to *kapha*, because immediately after entering the stomach, it strikes at the very root cause of vitiation of *kapha* [by acting to cleanse the stomach contents] and when it is overcome in the stomach, even the entire vitiated *kapha* dwelling in other parts of the body is automatically alleviated.[136]

So even though the site of the excess is the stomach, the site of the symptoms is the respiratory passage in the head: excess phlegm and blocked nasal passages. To go to the source (the stomach) and treat the cause, emetic therapy is given to cleanse the origin of the excess mucus.[137]

The Hippocratic physician had in mind the same process when he prescribed his emesis therapy. His was not a simplistic approach. Emesis was not the first part of the treatment. Rather the patient was carefully prepared for it by steps one to three. In this way it could have its maximum effect. The physician was 'leading' the separated humour to its proper site for final elimination, as in *Epidemics* 2.3, the material of apostases are led.[138]

Finally, we note food intake is to be reduced by half the next day. This seems to imply there was no food taken on the fourth day of treatment (that of the vomiting) and that it was only gradually increased back to the normal amount. In this way the imbalanced body, where food overpowered exercise (or the use of the food as fuel) is brought back into balance.

---

136. Sharma and Dash (1995) vol. I 371. Sūtrasthāna XX, 19.
137. Compare Hippocrates: "One must approach the cause, and of the cause, the source." *Epidemics*, 2.5 Smith (1994) 73.
138. Smith (1994) 57.

With regard to fasting, or abstaining from food, this is held by both Hippocratic medicine and by Āyurveda as a valid form of therapy, when undertaken at the right time and place and in the right circumstances according to the patient's constitution. In Āyurveda, as in Hippocratic medicine, physicians recognise the phenomenon that when the stomach is allowed a short rest from food digestion, certain effects can be seen to take place. One of these is that energy is released from the digestive process for use in other bodily processes. Another is that the bowels are allowed more time to empty completely, a desirable outcome. Finally, according to Āyurveda, the digestive fire, *agni* is actually increased in power so that when food comes next to be consumed, it will be better digested and thus better assimilated by the tissues.

By these therapeutic procedures in both Hippocratic and Ayurvedic medicine, the phlegmatic humour is caused to return to its normal state of *krasis* vis-a-vis the other humours.

## Pañcakarma or Therapeutic Cleansing in Āyurveda

An ancient five-fold cleansing treatment employing emesis, purging and others, is still being employed today in the treatment called '*pañca karma*' or five therapeutic actions. Athough it would not be used during acute disease, it would be employed after the patient had recovered, in order to restore balance and thoroughly cleanse the body. When medicinal measures have not brought about a balancing of the *doṣas*, this five-fold cleansing treatment is carried out. It consists first of a preparatory fast. Next two preparatory treatments are given, oleation or *snehana* (oiling the body to liquify and prepare the stagnant humour for removal), and sweating therapy *svedan* (to open the pores, warm the body and draw the toxins into the circulation for dispersal). These are followed by cleansing of the nasal passages; the small intestine with purgative herbs which remove *ama* and take it to the lower bowel for removal; the colon with enemas of medicinal herbs; emesis and blood letting (rarely used but now often substituted with blood cleansing herbs).[139]

139. See Sūtrasthāna, XIII-XV for basis of *pañcha karma.*

Recently, at a contemporary Ayurvedic clinic, a patient complaining of pains in the joints and being overweight, but who was not eating sufficiently was described as having a pattern of *"āmavat"*. *Ama* from the stomach had lodged in the joints along with excess *vāta* causing the pain. The patient was first prescribed a one-month course of oral herbal medicines and self-massage treatment with medicinal oils; dietary advice was also given. If these did not resolve the conditions, the doctor stated, the patient would then be advised to undergo the oleation and sweating therapy aspects of *pañca karma*.[140]

Holistic medicine today also emphasizes the importance of good quality of food and proper cooking and digestion for proper assimilation. The discipline of nutritional therapy recognises and works with the healing of disease through food and nourishment. Herbal traditions typically also put great emphasis on both a healthy diet for prevention of disease and maintenance of health, and also special diets, enemas, bowel cleansing and fasting as therapeutic strategies.[141] The basic theory and practice of Hippocratic medicine in acute diseases is evident in the practice of some contemporary herbalists and naturopaths. Therapeutic fasting and cleansing regimes, allied to herbal treatment, are a feature of herbalists trained by The School of Natural Healing (Provo, Utah), The School of Natural Medicine (Boulder, Colorado), The Holistic Health College (London) and The East-West College of Herbalism (Sussex, England).

## CONCLUSION

This chapter has examined the holistic approach of the Hippocratic physicians to disease as it is seen to originate in an imbalance in the digestive tract. It has explored in detail conditions

140. Observation in the clinic of Dr. Deepika Gunawant, 50 Penywern Road, London, May 23, 1996.

141. See the methods of Dr. John Christopher, and his students Michael Tierra and Farida Sharan in the West. Reference: *The School of Natural Healing, The Way of Herbs, Herbs of Grace*, respectively.

such as acute fever and catarrh. We have found that in many treatises, holistic ideas are indeed paramount. These include:

1. The attunement of assessment and treatment to the individual and engaging the individual in his or her own recovery.
2. The awareness of the mutual interaction between bodily and mental–emotional–spiritual experience and the choosing of therapy based on this awareness.
3. The awareness of the human organism as part of the larger cosmological environment and the incorporation of all such relevant information in assessment and treatment. This is primarily through the concepts of *pepsis* and *krasis*. Implicit in these are innate, vital heat, moisture and breath.

By incorporating a comparison of Hippocratic methods with those of Āyurveda as found in *Caraka*, we have been able to establish several areas of striking similarity and have been able to demonstrate that the Hippocratic approach, particularly such methods as therapeutic fasting, internal cleansing and dietary therapy, far from being merely a comforting treatment which was at least not harmful, comprises a sophisticated and carefully thought out programme, based on practical experience, not only to rid the body of disease but to return it to a positive state of well-being.

The information from *Caraka* has shed new light on one aspect of the Hippocratic approach which formerly may have been misunderstood, therefore neglected: the concept of therapeutic effects being based to a significant extent on the taste of the food/drug. I believe the disagreements and different approaches found in the treatises on the question of *dunameis*, whether it be a taste, a temperature or an effect, seems to suggest that this was a period when the physicians were learning more about their *materia medica* and attempting different ways of explaining the effects they were experiencing. The model in *Caraka* shows that physicians in ancient India may have been doing the same thing and that they did finally come up with concepts that allowed them to explain and organise the use of the many different therapeutic effects they found in food and herbal drugs.

CHAPTER 4

# HOLISM IN THE CONCEPT OF HUMOURS

The previous chapter examined the Hippocratic concepts of digestion and compared them to those of Āyurveda, finding that both traditions identify poor food, and poor digestion as an important cause of disturbance to the body's inherent balance, and thus of disease, through the creation of residues which accumulate and block the healthy processes in the body. An important component in whether the digestion and therefore health is balanced is the presence of proper coction.

A significant proportion of the Hippocratic treatises concentrate on diet and dietary therapy as the explanation for disease and means of recovering health. Yet another concept is equally characteristic of Greek medicine, that of the humours. This chapter examines this concept in the Hippocratic writings and the corresponding concept of tridoṣa, the three *doṣas,* in Āyurveda. The types of treatments chosen to carry out the humoural diagnosis will also be considered. An attempt will be made to pin-point what the humours meant to physicians of the day, as represented in the treatises. The fact that the authors of the dietary treatises also make reference to humours as factors or causes of health and disease, and to such other factors as seasons and weather, would indicate that the concept of humours in some form was also present in the approach of these physicians and that these two causes, diet and humours, were seen to be intertwined or mutually influential. The two concepts are further linked through the concept of coction which affects both.

From the point of view of comparative medicine, several Western scholars have noted the striking similarities between the two systems on this topic. Sigerist did not see similarities in the philosophical influences on medicine in the two ancient cultures, but notes that "we shall find great similarities in the procedures and achievements of Greek and Indian doctors."[1] Onians has also noted several examples of strong similarities between ancient Greek and Indian beliefs about aspects of the body and the soul.[2] Filliozat has given the most thorough examination of the question in recent times.[3] An important point of interest for some has been the question of whether there was influence from one tradition on the other. Filliozat argues that there was ample opportunity for cross-cultural exchanges in the centuries before Alexander's expedition to India in the fourth century B.C., mediated via the Persian empire and thus an exchange is highly probable. But there is no concrete evidence for any such transmission or influence.[4] This question is not the one being addressed in the present work.

Here the interest is rather to illuminate some aspects of Greek humoural concepts by comparison to the related concept of *doṣas* in Āyurveda, a holistic medicinal system in which *doṣas* are of the first importance in terms of diagnosis and treatment. This system is still being practised with success today. As discussed in Chapter One, both cultures show a major shift in outlook about the relationship of man and the cosmos in the century previous to that of Hippocratic writings. In each culture a new paradigm is established to explain phenomena, one based on reasoning from observation of nature, rather than on assumptions about the activities of deities or demons.

Most work on the humours as has been by classical scholars who, on the whole, have not taken seriously the humoural

1. Sigerist (1987) 182.
2. Onians (1994) 75, 196, 359-361.
3. Filliozat (1964).
4. West (1971) believes there was a period of active Iranian influence on the Greeks in the realm of philosophical–magical–religious ideas mediated through the Persian empire, which subsequently ceased. Sedlar (1980) points to common Indo–European roots (similar word origins, uses of chariots, similarities of deities), but says by the Homeric period Greeks confused India and Ethiopia. Filliozat (1964) 228-237, 257.

concepts in the *Corpus* as a realistic or effective means of diagnosis or therapeutics, although this has shown signs of changing in recent years.[5] The attempt here is to look afresh at the material without such assumptions because from the point of view of a holistic system such as Āyurveda, the rationale and the therapeutics of the system are of such similarity that they in fact can be seen to make sense. It is hoped that by approaching writings on humours in the *Corpus* from a point of view of a related system—one with its origins in the same era—the Hippocratic concepts may be more fully understood and appreciated.

## THE HIPPOCRATIC VIEW OF HUMOURS

A reader not trained in Classics coming to the *Corpus* and looking for a fundamentally unified explanation of the causes of disease and an exposition of the humoural concept and its application in practice may be disappointed and a little bewildered. There is a diversity of views on the causes of disease. *Anonymus Londinensis*, a late fifth century B.C. text that aims to record the views on the causes of disease by various physicians, also confirms this. If we read the treatises individually, we may be forgiven for being at a loss to find much common ground. Some mention humours quite specifically, some use the term apparently synonymously with 'elements' or constituents, some focus on tastes, others write only of the qualities hot, cold, wet, and dry. Some texts mention none of these.

This may not be so surprising when we recall that the *Corpus* is not a body of work by a single author or even a single redactor, nor does it reflect the approach of a single 'school'. Yet, there is common to the treatises what Jones terms a 'general pathology' which underlies the apparent diversity: the humoural model of health and disease.[6] Robert Joly, too, finds there is a fund of

5. See for example Lloyd (1987) 16: physicians deployed "pathological notions that were in, in many cases, entirely superficial". Compare Nutton, *Companion Encyclopedia of the History of Medicine*, (1993) vol.1, 281-291; Potter (1995) Introduction to translation of *Fleshes*, 129-130.
6. Jones (1981) vol. II 59.

doctrine common to the whole collection from which the writers draw.[7] Even the treatises that concentrate more on diet–digestion and dietary therapy as the cause of or means to disease and health, mention the constitutional types of phlegmatic and bilious, thus acknowledging the humoural background to their approach.[8]

Among the apparent diversity and argumentation there is important common ground. Firstly, the concepts of cooking, mingling, harmony[9] ; secondly, the humoural model or models. Each of these represent rational ways of explaining the human body. Finally, underpinning these and all the works in the *Corpus* and providing a unifying framework is, as Thivel and Jouanna point out, the fact that their explanations focus on man within the wider cosmological context: the same laws which can be seen to govern and regulate universal natural phenomena of the larger, non-biological world, particularly as regards change and transformation.[10] For example, the process of evaporation, the nature of fire, of cold and of ice, all such phenomena are understood to be at work within all living things, including man. There is a 'transference' of this understanding from the outer cosmos to the biological sphere which represents a unity of view: that man is the microcosm within the macrocosm.

One can also add that it is a very practical transference to the human sphere, as both Sigerist and Lloyd point out.[11] For while philosophers are concerned with the origins and nature of existence in general and of the larger natural world, and man's ultimate being, physicians have to deal with the day-to-day realities of helping the sick, of trying to relieve their suffering. But to help in this effort, they also seek to know and understand both the nature of the world at large and the particular nature of man, and the interactions between these two.

---

7. Joly (1975) 122 and 127.
8. See for example, *Ancient Medicine*.
9. *pepsis, kresis, harmonia*.
10. Thivel (1981) 306. Jouanna (1988) Introduction to *Vents*, 26.
11. Sigerist (1987) 318 "Force and quality were rather vague concepts...the physicians looked for more tangible substances which could explain the phenomena of health and disease." Lloyd (1986) 42.

## The Nature of Man is Humoural

In Chapter Two attention was drawn to the regard for the importance of nature as the fundamental, creative life principle among the Hippocratic physicians. In addition to the universal nature, as Lain Entralgo has pointed out, there was for the ancient Greeks also an individual *phusis*, the nature of the individual, particular to each man and his parts.[12] This individual nature is naturally the main concern of the physicians, as several treatises testify. What man is made of, and how he interacts with his environment, and even, in some treatises, with his internal or what we now call his subconscious or spiritual self. This may be more the point of the polemic of some authors against philosophers or others who speak of 'the hot, the cold' than that they are, as proto-scientists, somehow rebelling against their philosophical context. The physician–author of *Ancient Medicine* points out that he is primarily interested in what constitutes and influences a man. This does not, however, mean he totally dissociates himself from the 'philosophical', despite what he says in chapter XX. For although he states that "all that philosophers or physicians have said or written on natural science no more pertains to medicine than to painting," he also "hold[s] that clear knowledge about natural science can be acquired from medicine and from no other source....I mean...what man is, by what causes he is made and similar points...this at least I think a physician must know...what man is *in relation to* foods and drinks and to habits generally and what will be the effects of each on each individual." [emphasis mine]. He values and seeks the same knowledge, but relies on the disciplines of medicine, not of other philosophers, for this knowledge. The author of *Nature of Man* similarly distances himself from the philosophers:

> I do not say at all that man is air, or fire, or water, or earth or anything else that is not an obvious constituent of man.(I)[13]

---

12. Lain Entralgo (1970) 145-147.
13. Jones (1979) vol. IV 3.

yet his model of humours as the constituents of man still relates them to the cosmos at large, to seasons, and climates.

The author of *Regimen I* similarly cites the importance of knowing "the nature of man in general,...from what things he is originally composed and discern by what parts he is controlled" (II).[14] Thus these physicians apparently agreed on the primary importance of knowing 'what man is', but preferred to derive the answer more specifically from their own sphere, medicine, rather than relying on the testimony from philosophy. Drawing this distinction may have been part of their efforts to establish a higher status for their craft within the society. Other works in the *Corpus* do not strive for such distinction from philosophy. An example is *Nutriment*, a Heraclitean work which reproduces the master's aphoristic style.[15] And it is possible that there was a kind of guild or brotherhood among some physicians who worked from their own metaphysical or religious discipline.[16] But whether they distinguished themselves, their remaining writings reflect the fact that they were concerned to apply any such knowledge to the practicalities of treating individuals. Since man is part of the cosmos at large, the transference enables them to apply to human experience the observations derived from the natural world. *Disease I*, 2 states directly that

> Bile and phlegm come into being with man's coming into being, and are always present in the body in greater or lesser amounts. They produce diseases, however, partly because of the effects of food and drinks, and partly as the result of heat that makes them too hot, or cold that makes them too cold.[17]

Iain Lonie's discussion of the humoural theory seems to sense this situation. In *The Hippocratic Treatises "On Generation and On the Nature of the Child, Diseases IV*, Lonie argues, based on

14. Ibid., 227.
15. Jones (1972) vol. I 337.
16. The Hippocratic Oath and the treatise *Law* suggest this. Edelstein (1967), Jones (1981) 258.
17. Potter (1988) vol. V 103. This passage seems to sum up the varieties of ideas on humours, relating them to foods, to excess deficiencies, and to heat and cold.

the evidence of *Nature of Man* and *Ancient Medicine*, that though physicians rejected "the application to medicine of specific cosmological doctrines...they accept, perhaps unconsciously, the general intellectual framework."[18] He says that for the identification of those things that make up man, they turned to their own traditions and found there "well-established, the concept of bodily humours...the humours became the constituent elements of the human body."[19] This would be a kind of annexation of the concept of constituent elements from philosophy to the humours and thus marks a significant change, or development in the traditional concept of a 'humour'. Unfortunately, while Lonie discusses the nature of these humours, he does not elucidate this previous tradition from which the physicians drew their 'own' tradition. Was this tradition medical or something else?

Since there are no specifically medical writings prior to the fifth century, we cannot establish a previous specifically medical tradition. In pre-literate societies still existing today there is a vast knowledge of effective healing practices and plants in folk traditions or popular consciousness. It would seem probable that such was the basis of a certain amount of Hippocratic practice. Ann Ellis Hanson indicates that the recipes in the gynaecological works preserve elements of an oral tradition among women.[20] This suggests, though is not concrete proof of, such a folk tradition from which the physicians drew their terms. Similarly Thivel feels that in many ways the physicians appropriated pre-existing popular ideas and used them for their own purposes. He discusses two layers of tradition in the *Corpus*, an older Ionian one and a newer one from the fourth century B.C.[21]

Evidence of such a tradition about humours is given to some extent in *The Origins of European Thought* by R.B. Onians. Although Onians does not investigate the humours, phlegm or melancholy, he documents the expressions in literature of

18. Lonie (1981) 56.
19. Ibid.
20. Hanson (1990) 310.
21. Thivel (1981) 306-307.

various kinds relating particularly to bile, the liver and blood and also to other concepts found in the *Corpus* such as the soul, the vital breath, vital moisture and the nature of the contents of the brain and the vital spinal marrow.[22] In particular the physical fluid bile relates to the emotion anger and affects the way men think and behave. Disturbances to blood also disturb thought. Melancholy as a normal healthy bodily humour is perhaps more difficult to understand as, before the treatise *Nature of Man*, it was mainly found as a common term for abnormal mental states, or madness.[23] (This issue is discussed below on page 191.) Thivel believes that the mental–spiritual aspects of both bile and melancholy were appropriated by the physicians from popular thought.[24] The ideas about bodily humours, the linking of physical fluids with mental–emotional states predates the *Corpus* and the physicians accepted these and made use of them in their understanding of 'what man is'.

## Medical Reasoning

While in one sense partaking of traditional views, the physicians also sought to distinguish themselves from them in other areas. They wished to develop a model for medical practice. According to Lain Entralgo in *The Therapy of the Word in Classical Antiquity*, the physicians established a particular *logismos iatrikos* or way of reasoning, a way of "explaining what reality 'is'", for their craft.[25] This had to be faithful to the *logos* (truth, reality) of the *phusis*, the truth about nature, and physicians were trained not be misled by appearances. Since nature was both human

---

22. Onians (1994). For *psuche* as a *daimon* surviving death, see p. 118; as something gaseous and an originator of movement, see p. 165; as informing spirit in the fluid see p. 196. For breath–oul or consciousness in the *thumos*, see pp. 44-60. For consciousness connected to bile, the liver and feelings, see pp. 84-87; as connected to the brain and spinal marrow, see pp.118.; as connected to the thigh bone, see pp. 182, 205-206, n. 5. For marrow as vehicle for seed, see pp. 115. For vital fluids see pp. 210-215; for moisture as vehicle for seed, see pp. 202-203.
23. Sigerist (1961) 333, n. 8 He is relying on Walter Muri's 'Melancholie und schwarze Galle', Museum Helveticum 1953, 10 p. 34f.
24. Ibid. 316, 312.
25. Lain Entralgo (1970) 148, 151.

and divine, aiming to know the truth about man to a certain extent included aiming to know the truth about universal truths. Their medical reasoning distinguished physicians' medicine from other healers', such as temple medicine and charm sellers and defined the basis of their *techne*. As Lain Entralgo translates from *Places in Man*, 6: "the *phusis* of the body is the principle/*arche* of the logos in medicine". He goes on,

> That is, the nature of the human body is the reality to which the *logos* of the physician should above all be applied.[26]

This shows that for physicians, medicine involves both practical skills and a philosophical perspective through which to evaluate, organise and treat bodily phenomena.

But this philosophical perspective did not abstract them from their context. Their art was still very much part of the wider *milieu*. Physicians were in contact with all classes of society, attending both slaves and free, male and female. They were in contact with midwives and prostitutes,[27] priests, the poor and the rich; and they were present at *symposia* to expound on the medical point of view the subject being discussed.

Medical reasoning would also give them a means of, or basis for, formulating and applying their therapy. It was the way of organising and above all interpreting the information available to them from their visual, tactile, olfactory, taste and aural observations of their patients. Acute observations were necessary, but at the same time,

> the wise man should prefer his intelligence to his eyes if he is trying to know what things are under the mantle of their immediate appearance.[28]

26. Lain Entralgo (1970) 148.
27. Prostitutes are mentioned in Potter (1995) 161, and Lonie (1978), in Lloyd (1986) 325. Indications are that physicians derived much of their knowledge of women's diseases, of childbirth and early infancy from women. Elements of their oral tradition are preserved in the recipes of the gynaecological treatises. Hanson (1990) 310.
28. Ibid., 149. Lain Entralgo quotes from *Regimen I*, V: "More trust is placed in the eyes than in the intelligence, when they are not sufficient even to discern what they see. For my part I ask explanation of the intelligence." He cites *The Art*, and *Law* for the physicians' awareness of the contrast between conventions and spontaneous reality of things, and of the products of right and true *logos*, and the products of fleeting and superficial *logos*.

A good physician does not take observations at face value, as an untrained or poorly trained person might do. *Ancient Medicine* XXI states that "most physicians, like laymen...[are] ignorant of the real cause" of a disturbance. *The Art* XIV speaks of "interpreting the information before it can be utilised by medical intelligence." The best physicians then obtain from reasoning and inference a discernment of the state of affairs within the body. Further, when they apply these reasonings, they find they can get results. They can influence the body in such a way as to restore health in many cases. Applying their medical reasoning they can also tell which clients they can help and those who are beyond their help, thus it is also the basis of the art of *prognostikon.*[29]

What the medical practitioners of the fifth and fourth centuries seem to have done is to combine traditional concepts of humours and healing techniques based on centuries of empirical experience with their more recently developed skills of medical reasoning about man's nature which linked the microcosm to the macrocosm. Their method was now disengaged from theocentric thought though not from awareness of the divine. It enabled them to explain to themselves the phenomena they were witnessing in their ill and healthy clients.

## The Meaning of 'Humours'

Even before the physicians took up the ideas of elements and humours these concepts were established in popular consciousness derived from observation and experience. The term humour comes ultimately from the root *cheo*: to pour, melt, dissolve, spread. Hence it refers to a liquid. Other forms of this root give: juice, moisture, the extracted flavour, or taste (*chulos, chumos*). The term was used in connection with plants, i.e. their saps or tastes, and with processes, such as melting, dissolving, spreading. It also was used to indentify aspects of the human body,

29. Jones (1972) vol. I 57 and (1981) vol. II. 217. Compare *iatrikon logikon* with the very similar *yukti*, which, as described by Chattopadhyaya (1979) 207, usually means 'rational application' but in the medical text it refers to the intellectual discipline or technique of determining how a number of factors jointly produce a special effect. See also 391.

such as tastes, tissues and bodily fluids. This last meaning, fluid or fluid secretions, is the most common use of the term in the *Corpus*, and the most commonly understood meaning, especially relating to the fluids bile and phlegm. The aspect of *cheo* which relates to melting, dissolving and spreading also may be significant for the humoural model of health-disease-treatment, as will be discussed below.

For the Greeks, humours represented the very physical manifestation of certain fundamental and necessary vital principles, without which the body would not be what it is. If we consider that the living body is characterised above all by warmth along with a certain amount of dryness, by moisture and movement, and also by consciousness, then these qualities become the vital ones. If present in abnormal amounts (excess or deficiency) they may also become threats to life.

One of these principles necessary to life, since its absence is most obvious in death, is that of innate heat.[30] Another is that of the breath–soul consciousness dwelling in the body's *thumos* (chest region) as a moist vapour. Moisture is also embodied as the vital sap or fluid, the very stuff of life and of strength and also the vehicle for procreation. In the body this vital sap resides in the brain or encephalon and in the spinal marrow or cerebral spinal fluid; by extension, through the spinal fluid it exists in the marrow of the bones themselves, and in the generative fluid.

## Humours as Fundamental Constituent Elements

The answer the physicians give to their question of the nature of man is that he is composed, fundamentally, of these vital essences as humours. Thivel discusses how the bi-polarity of phlegm and bile represent an older tradition, where the humours derive from the elements of fire and water.[31] *Regimen I*, III actually recognises that the elemental principles themselves are in the body:

30. Onians (1951) 46, 95, and n. 5, Jones (1981) 217 (*The Art* XIV) for *thermotera*, (1979) 105, (*Aphorisms* I, XIV) for *thermon*.
31. Thivel (1981) 305-306.

> Now all animals, including man, are composed of two things, different in power but working together in their use, namely, fire and water. Both together these are sufficient for one another and for everything else, but each by itself suffices neither for itself nor for anything else.

(This may be the kind of thinking that the author of *Ancient Medicine* was opposed to.) For most of the writers, the qualities of the elements are manifested in the body as the humours.[32]

The physicians of course recognise there are other things that are found in the body so can be said to be part of man; individual tissues, organs and structures, for example, are also discussed in the treatises and are locations for diseases. There seems to be some overlap between the concepts of humour and of tissue. For example, the blood comes to be considered a humour, though not a secreted fluid in the same sense as bile and phlegm. And even though the author of *Ancient Medicine* seems to prefer tastes—acrid, pungent, bitter, astringent, sweet—as constituents and diseases factors, as we have seen (XIV, XV) he certainly evidently bases his practice, at least partly, on humours for he states,

> I hold that it is also necessary to know which diseased states arise from powers and which from structures. What I mean is roughly that a power is an intensity and strength of the humours, while structures are conformations to be found in the human body... (XXII).[33]

In fact, the taste principles are identified with the humours in chapter XIX, which is understandable if we recall that nouns derived from *cheo* can mean either fluid or savour/taste, so that ultimately for this writer disease is attributed to imbalance in humours.[34]

---

32. Ibid., 316. Thivel speaks of the "transformation of the humours 'being' of the elements of the spirit into the physical cause of disease".
33. Jones (1972) vol. I 57.
34. By contrast Smith seems to think that *Nature of Man* and *Ancient Medicine* cannot be 'reconciled'. Smith (1979) 22.

Whether they be one (the air or *aither* of Anaximenes), two (the fire and water of Heraclitus), three, four (the 'roots' of Empedocles) or more, in essence the humours represent a transference of the cosmological elements to the body, both as fluids and as bodily constituents in the sense of actual tissues or organs. (*Fleshes*, for example, discusses how the different body structures are formed from the elements.) In the sense that without them, the body would not be as it is, would not exist, they are the basic constituent or constituting elements and are normal and healthy. To the extent that these necessary constituents become imbalanced, they are the causes of disease, abnormal and destructive to life.[35]

## Humoural Models

In the *Corpus*, though the basic qualities and characteristics of the humours are common to all, we find different ideas as to how many humours are important and how they are organised.

The most prominent humours in the *Corpus* are phlegm and bile. Sometime it is simple bile and phlegm that are discussed, sometimes they are differentiated: for example, a white phlegm is mentioned and bile is sometimes distinguished as yellow, acid, or bitter. Bile is normally heating and drying (fire), phlegm while in itself being cooling and moistening (water), when it is imbalanced (excessive or congested) it can provoke heat or fevers (e.g. *The Sacred Disease*).

*Fleshes* does not speak of humours but does discuss the constituents of man, how his body is formed according to a tri-polar model of the elements and qualities: *aither* (heat), earth (dryness) and an intervening atmosphere (moisture). Some treatises mention additional body components or fluids as humours : blood (*Nature of Man*), water (*Diseases IV*), black bile (*Nature of Man, Epidemics 4, Diseases IV*).

35. Lonie (1981) 57-58.

The eventual identification of four cardinal humours that we find in *Nature of Man* and *Diseases IV* is considered as a later development. *Nature of Man* is thought to incorporate the four root elements of Empedocles, fire, earth, air and water,[36] but it could also be that other factors were influencing the physicians as will be suggested below.

## Sites and Movements of Humours

In addition to being seen as present everywhere in the body, humours were also associated with certain main sites. In the treatise *Disease IV* the four humours are explicitly considered to be sited in a specific organ: the head for phlegm, the heart for blood, the gall-bladder for bile and the spleen for water. Each humour is also seen to be present in food, something from the external environment, and when food is digested, each 'reservoir' attracts to itself primarily its related humour, though subsequently others as well. (The exception is the gall-bladder, whose narrow vessels can accommodate only bile. Here it is stored so that it can be imparted to the body if and when the humour becomes diminished in it.) Equilibrium of humours throughout the body is thus maintained.[37] The humours are thus strongly linked to the digestive tract and digestive processes, as well as to individual reservoir sites.

A humour can move from its site when it becomes imbalanced (excessive, congested). This is allowed for, as Lonie has pointed out, by empty space, or void.[38] This features prominently in the model of *Diseases IV* and *Nature of the Child* to explain the movement of humours (and the growth of the embryo) since an empty space attracts matter to fill it, both like and unlike.[39] Lonie believes this to be "the key to the whole humoural theory." This concept is especially interesting in comparison with Ayurveda which, we recall, also recognises the importance of space *(ākāśa)* as one of the five cosmic elements.

---

36. Lonie (1981) 61.
37. Ibid., *Diseases IV*, 33-41 and commentary by Lonie 260.
38. *euruxorin*.
39. Ibid., 266.

Before considering the nature of the humours and their characteristics in more detail, let us briefly survey the corresponding concepts about dosas in the Ayurvedic tradition.

## THE CONCEPT OF TRIDOṢA IN *CARAKA SAṂHITĀ*

In spite of some differences, the model of three humours, tridoṣa, is in several aspects strikingly similar to those of the *Corpus*. As was discussed in Chapter One, Āyurveda was forming as a rational medical system during a period of philosophical interest in the nature of the physical world similar to that which occurred in the Greek world in the fifth and sixth centuries. The Ayurvedic physicians made use of philosophical concepts from several 'schools' of thought when forming their system. The most prominent among these are the Vaiśeṣika and the Sāṃkhya. Explanations from both are found in *Caraka* (e.g. Sūtrasthāna I) but that of Sāṃkhya is discussed more fully. Most scholars think that what is represented in *Caraka* is a mixture from different periods gathered together in the second century text that is preserved for us. Taking the text as it is, we find the following concepts:[40]

As outlined in Chapter Two, from an eternal, unmanifested 'absolute soul' the creation is manifested through five great elements or *pañcamahābhūta.* (Śārīrasthāna I, verses 60-64)[41] Each element is further also explicitly associated with certain qualities, attributes, or characteristics both in the natural world and in the individual human:

*Ākāśa* : aether space, full of an extremely rarefied substance and having the attribute of sound,

*Vāyu* : wind or air has the attributes of sound plus touch and the characteristic of motion,

*Tejas* : fire has attributes of sound, touch plus vision and the characteristic of heat,

*Jala* : water has attributes of sound, touch, vision plus taste and the characteristic of liquidity, and

*Pṛthvī* : earth has attributes of sound, touch, vision, taste plus smell and the characteristic of roughness.[42]

---

40. I am indebted to Anne Glazier for these clarifications.
41. Sharma and Dash (1994) vol. II 327.
42. Ibid., 318-319.

## Elements form *Doṣas*

In the microcosm of the human body these elements, with their qualities combine in various ways to form the three *doṣas* and the seven *dhātus* or tissues. The three *doṣas* are *vāta, pitta* and *kapha.* As in the Hippocratic treatises, an explicit definition or explanation of the exact constitution and origin of a *doṣa* is not given in *Caraka.* The three doṣas are said to be responsible for the maintenance of the health of the individual (Sūtrasthāna XII, 13),[43] and so the wise endeavour to keep them in their normal state (Śārīrasthāna VI, 18).[44] At the same time, they are referred to as the causative factors in diseases (Sūtrasthāna I, verse 57).[45] The term *doṣa* itself does literally mean 'fault' and is used not only to refer to basic bodily constituents. It carries with it the idea of defect or weakness, thus, while they are natural to the body, the doṣas are also the means by which disease – or dis-harmony – is caused when they become imbalanced.

The term *dhātu* is also used when discussing the composition of the body. The Sanskrit term *dhātu* is used in many contexts. It can mean a layer or stratum; a constituent part, ingredient or element; and primitive matter itself. It can refer to the grammatical root or stem, the basic element, as of a word and also to a primary element as of earth, that is, an ore. It also is used in describing the human body. It appears to have two meanings in the text of *Caraka.*

The first is a distinct meaning as the tissues elements of the body—also derived from the mahābhūtas (Śārīrasthāna VI, 4).[46] These are seven: the 'food or chyle-juice'/*rasa*, blood/*rakta*, flesh/*māṃsa*, fat/*medas*, bone/*asthi*, marrow/*majjan* and semen or reproductive fluid/*śukra.* There is also an additional special substance in the body termed *ojas* which is the essential vital fluid. The second meaning of *dhātu* is close to that of *doṣa*, in the sense that a state of equilibrium of the tissue elements is

43. Ibid., vol. I 242.
44. Ibid., vol. II 440.
45. Ibid., vol. I 41 Mental factors or gunas as also mentioned in this verse.
46. Ibid., vol. II 427.

health and when a tissue element becomes diseased it is a factor in the disease process and is treated as such (Śārīrasthāna VI, verse 4; I, verses 86-94).[47] The two terms are in fact sometimes used interchangeably and sometimes distinguished (Sūtrasthāna XVII, 17, 63-72).[48] Julius Jolly explains that

> The usual name *doṣa* (defect) shows that *doṣas* deranged or existing in excess are to be properly treated. The name *dhātu* characterises them as the elements of the body.[49]

The authoritative commentator Cakrapāṇidatta also has noted this interchangeability. He says that

> *'doṣas'* include *'dhātus'* and vice-versa. So the drugs that are designated as alleviators of the dosas also alleviate *dhatus*. Similarly the drugs that have been designated as vitiators of the *dhatus* do as well vitiate doṣas.[50]

Anne Glazier, a Sanskrit scholar currently working on the medical texts, believes that what this may represent is the combining of two strands of traditions, yet to be completely harmonised.[51]

Blood, *rakta dhātu*, appears to have a special importance. Cakrapāṇidatta's commentary on Sūtrasthāna I, 57 points out that

> it is not that the pathogenic factors are confined only to *vāta, pitta, kapha*....A mention about *rakta*—its specific causes of vitiation, signs, symptoms of vitiation, diseases due to its vitiation and treatment is also made in...Sūtrasthāna XXIV, 9, 18, 22. Thus apparently *rakta* is also treated as one of the pathogenic factors and so there should be a fourfold classification of such factors instead of three. But the reason why *rakta* has not been included in the classification of pathogenic factors is that this is not

47. Ibid., 427 and 335.
48. Ibid., vol. I 303, 322-324.
49. Jolly (1994) 49.
50. Sharma and Dash (1994) vol. I 49. Cakrapāṇidatta is the author of an eleventh century commentary on *Caraka*, which is considered to be most authoritative. His commentary is included alongside the translation of *Caraka* in the edition being used for the purposes of this book.
51. Interview, June, 1997.

> in itself an independent pathogenic factor. It is so only when it is vitiated by *vāta, pitta*, or/and *kapha*. *Vāta, pitta, kapha*, unlike *rakta*, constitute independent pathogenic factors.[52]

Muelenbeld has also commented that although the Ayurvedic model is usually said to have three *doṣas*, in fact, blood, otherwise a *dhātu* or tissue, is sometimes spoken of as if it were a fourth humour.[53]

The same *mahābhūtas* are manifested in nature at large and in the human body, so that aspects of the natural world can be used to understand and treat diseases. This explains the useful actions of *dravyas*, the drugs or material substances used for treatments (Sūtrasthāna I, verses 63-68).[54] Thus curable diseases may be cured by using drugs of the opposite qualities to those of the imbalanced *doṣa* (verses 59-63).[55] The specific qualities of the *doṣas* are as follows:

> The qualities of *vāta* are: rough, cool, light, subtle, mobile, 'un-unctuous' or dry, quick, abundant in quantity, and coarse.
> The qualities of *pitta* are: unctuous, hot sharp, liquid, sour, fluid and pungent.
> The qualities of *kapha* are: heavy, cool, soft, unctuous, sweet, immobile and slimy (Sūtrasthāna I, 59-60).[56]

These qualities derive ultimately from combinations of the qualities of the *mahābhūtas.* (Śārīrasthāna IV, 12) [57] *Kapha* combines *jalap* and *pṛthvī*. *Pitta* combines *tejas* and *jalap*. *Vāta* combines *ākāśa* and *vāyu.*

Each *doṣa* is said to be located in particular sites in the body. The colon is the most important site for *vāta*, but it is also located in the bladder, rectum, thighs, waist, legs, and bones. The small intestine (lower part) is the main site for *pitta*, but it is also located in tissues *rasa* and *rakta*, and in the waste material

---

52. Sharma and Dash (1994) vol. I 42.
53. Muelenbeld (1995) 4.
54. Sharma and Dash (1994) vol. I 45-50.
55. Ibid., 43-44.
56. Ibid., 43.
57. Ibid., vol. II 392 See also Sūtrasthāna I, 64 as explained by Cakrapāṇidatta's commentary. vol. I 45-46.

sweat. The chest is the main site of *kapha*, but it is also located in the stomach, head, neck, joints and the *medas*/fat tissue. At the same time, each *doṣa* also is present in all parts of the body (Sūtrasthāna XX, 8-9).[58] The digestive tract —the stomach, small intestine and colon—includes the main sites of two of the *doṣas*, *pitta* and *vāta*, and one of the sites of the third, *kapha*. This is important in the aetiology of diseases from poor food digestion. In the digestive process, these main sites of *doṣas* become imbalanced and from here the *doṣas* move into other areas of the body, through channels and into tissues. Such movement is also important for treatment because the aim of treatment is first to rebalance the state of deranged *doṣas* at these distant sites and then lead them back to their main sites, the excess to be eliminated through the elimination areas of the body: the nasal passages, mouth (vomiting and nasal cleansing), bowels (purgation, enema), skin (sweating therapy).

Although different parts of the body are made up of combinations of *doṣas*, one *doṣa* is responsible for a particular body function, organ or tissue. Thus *vāta* is responsible for all movement, co-ordination and regulation, auditory and tactile senses, and elimination of wastes. *Pitta* is responsible for digestion, vision and perception, metabolism in general, complexion, colour and pigmentation in the body, and bodily heat in general. *Kapha* is responsible for the strength and stability, clarity and softness of complexion, healthy state of the bodily fleshes and fluids in general (Sūtrasthāna XII, 8, 11, 12; XVII, 115-118 and Vimānasthāna VIII, 96, 97, 98).[59] At the same time, it is recognised that the *doṣas* mingle together throughout the body.

As well as *doṣas* in the physical make up of the body, two mental *doṣas* are mentioned (Śārīrasthāna, III, 13; IV, 34).[60] Sūtrasthāna, I verses 55-56 says that the body and mind constitute the substrata of diseases and happiness because the mahābhūtas also are part of the consciousness of the individual human, indeed enable this consciousness to perceive the physical

58. Ibid., vol. I 362.
59. Ibid., 239, 241; 335 and vol. II 263-266.
60. Ibid., vol. II 378-379; 405-406.

world through the senses.[61] Thus the same elemental factors that are part of the larger creation are also present and active in the individual human. Sūtrasthāna I, 46-47 states:

> mind, soul and body—these three are like a tripod; the world is sustained by their combination; they constitute the substratum for everything. This [combination] is *Puruṣa*." [the cosmic entity.[62]

Sūtrasthāna XII gives the characteristics of each *doṣa* in the body in its 'normal state', and specifically includes the mental-emotional aspects. For example, for *vāta* these are joy; for *pitta* valour, joy, and happiness; for *kapha*, enthusiasm, wisdom and peacefulness. Their opposites appear when the doṣa is imbalanced, e.g. fear, anger, laziness and ignorance.[63] Śārīrasthāna II, verse 40 also recognises the effect of the mind on the body when it states that disease can be caused by "intellectual blasphemy/ *prajñāparādha*, and unwholesome contact of the mind with the senses and seasonal vagaries."[64] Thus Āyurveda conceives of the human body as a psycho-physical whole, part of the wider creation, whose constitutional elements it shares. Or perhaps rather than human body, we should say human being, that energetic manifestation of the five subtle elements and inclusive of body, mind-emotions and higher consciousness, soul–spirit.

If the balance of the *doṣas* in the body is harmonious, there is health, if not disease is initiated (Vimānasthāna I, 5; Śārīrasthāna VI, 18).[65] There are three states of *doṣas*: normal (balanced and healthy), diminished (deficient) and aggravated (excessive) (Sūtrasthāna XVII, 112-114).[66] *Doṣas* are said to move in the body in three ways: upwards, downwards and sideways. They do so through the three channels: the central channel (digestive tract), the external channel (the more superficial tissues of the body, *rakta* and rasa), and the internal channel (the vital organs and functions)

---

61. Ibid., vol. I 40, 41.
62. Ibid., 33.
63. Ibid., 237, 240-241; see also Vimānasthāna VIII, verses 96-98 in vol. II 263-266.
64. Ibid., vol. II 362. See also Sūtrasthāna XI, 43 and XX, 5 vol. I; 226, 361.
65. Ibid., 113, 440.
66. Ibid., vol. I 333.

(Sūtrasthāna XVII, 112-114). *Doṣas* are also seasonal in nature, i.e. they accumulate, are aggravated and are alleviated in the six seasons.[67]

## The Stages of Disease

If the *doṣas* become imbalanced, they can cause disease through a series or stages of changes:

1. A *doṣa* accumulates to excess or gets diminished in its particular site, e.g. *vāta* has a tendency to accumulate to excess in the colon.
2. The *doṣa* is provoked or alleviated by a factor of like or opposite character, such as the season (Sūtrasthāna XVII, verse 114; Śārīrasthāna I, verses 110-112; Vimānasthāna VIII, passage 127),[68] foods, time of day, habitat or location. Or another *doṣa* can become mixed with it. It is usually not all, but only one or two of the qualities of a *doṣa* which aggravate those like qualities of another. For example, the cold of *kapha* can aggravate the cold of *vāta,* even though in other respects the two are quite opposite (Vimānasthāna VI, passage 10).[69]
3. A *doṣa*, or mixture of *doṣas,* which is excessive or diminished, is said to move through one of the three channels, or directions, possibly obstructing the channels. By means of the channels it spreads to vital organs (Sūtrasthāna XVII, verses 112-114).[70]
4. A *doṣa* can mix with another *doṣa,* with one or more of its qualities (Vimānasthāna VI, passage10),[71] or with *ama*, the residue of incomplete digestion (Vimānasthāna II, passage 7).[72]
5. At the new site (the organ or tissue), the *doṣa* can displace or obstruct another *doṣa* in its normal condition there, and the organ or tissue, causing problems and symptoms according to its qualities (Sūtrasthāna XVII, verses 41-61, 63-72).[73]

---

67. Ibid., 333.
68. Ibid., 333-334; vol. II 339; 283. For examples see Sūtrasthāna XVII, 11-40.
69. Ibid., vol. II 187.
70. Ibid., vol. I 333.
71. Ibid., vol. II 187.
72. Ibid., 134-135.
73. Ibid., 317-325.

An example of a *doṣa* affecting an organ would be that given to explain the *paittika* (*pitta* type) of heart disease. It is distinguished from a *kaphaja* (*kapha* type) or *vātika* (*vāta* type) because *pitta doṣa* has affected the heart. (The heart can also be affected by all three *doṣas* in imbalance, a worst-case scenario, Sūtrasthāna XVII, verses 30-36).[74] Cikitsāsthāna III, verses 129-132, describes the process of pathogenic changes in the case of fever:

> Three aggravated *doṣas*, either jointly or in combination of two or three, spread through the *rasa dhatu* and dislodge the digestive fire (*jaṭharāgni*) from its own place. Being supplemented with their own heat and the heat of the *jaṭharāgni*, the heat of the body gets accentuated. These channels of circulation get obstructed by them and they, being further aggravated, pervade the entire body to produce excessive heat.[75]

The qualities of the *doṣas* influence or determine the way the *doṣa* behaves in the body. For example, since *kapha* is heavy and cool, it tends to create sluggishness and accumulate in fleshy or fluid tissues, such as the nasal passages as catarrh. *Pitta* is light, mobile and hot and tends to affect the blood tissue. *Vāta* is cooling, drying and can easily become irregular; it tends to dry out tissues and affect the muscles and all movements (what we today would recognise as affecting nervous function or joints as in arthritis). Knowledge of these qualities means the ability to both understand, make sense of what is happening in the body, and to predict how the body may change given these conditions. Factors which imbalance or influence the state of the *doṣas* can come from any aspect of human experience; the body is intimately connected with both external forces of nature and the cosmos and internal processes and factors. Hence the body's state of health is affected from outside by the climate, seasons, place of living, type of work and exercise, type of food growing in the area; also from sudden traumatic events such as

74. Ibid., 316.
75. Ibid., vol. III 146.

poisoning or wounding. From inside ill health comes from disturbances of *doṣas*, or from the residues/*ama* produced from digestion which can clog the channels and mix with the *doṣas*. 'Internal' factors can also include past deeds or karmas from a previous life (since the effects of these are part of the consciousness of the individual and are influencing him).[76] The physician takes account of all these factors when assessing the patient (Sūtrasthāna XX, 20-25).[77]

## Individual Nature: *Prakṛti*

Such knowledge of numerous factors involved in an illness is also part of the concept of the individual *prakṛti* or constitutional nature of the patient. In Āyurveda, *prakṛti*, a term also found in Sāṃkhya philosophy, means both the physical creation or nature in general, and the particular nature or constitution of an individual human being: the way the *doṣas* are constituted in an individual, their balance vis-a-vis each other. Hence, there is an intimate relationship between the microcosm and the macrocosm:

> The individual is the epitome of the universe. All the material and spiritual phenomena of the universe are present in the individual. Similarly all those present in the individual are also contained in the universe. This is how the wise perceive (Śārīrasthāna IV, passage13).[78]

As this passage shows, the Ayurvedic physicians were well aware of the mind–body–spirit reality of their patients, and took this into account when understanding the diseases and formulating treatment. We have seen above that each doṣa represented the mental-emotional make-up—a predisposition to emotions such as fear or anger—as well as a purely physical one. In general, psychic aspects of the person's make-up are considered in the realm of the mind and the quality of the mind is determined by the three *guṇas*, or 'mental *doṣas*': *sattva* —

76. Ibid., vol. II 153. Life span is said to be influenced, though not completely determined by the past lives.
77. Ibid., vol. I 372-373.
78. Ibid., vol. II 393.

clear, peaceful, harmonious, *rajas*—active, disturbed and *tamas*—sluggish, inert, darkened. The latter two are called *doṣas* of the mind and are the ones which can disturb the somatic *doṣas* and initiate imbalance that causes disease (Śārīrasthāna IV, passage 34).[79] For example, in *Caraka* Nidānasthāna the causes of epilepsy (*apaśmara*) are given as five-fold: mind overshadowed by *rajas* and *tamas*, *doṣas* exceedingly aggravated and equilibrium disturbed, unclean or unwholesome food, or with mutually contradictory properties, unhealthy lifestyle and suffering excessive debility. The aggravated *doṣas* then permeate the heart—the abode par excellence of the soul and senses—and there are said to be disturbed by grief, anger, greed, fear, passion, excitement and anxiety (Nidānasthāna VIII, passage 4).[80]

In addition, there is evidence in *Caraka* that, although the physicians' approach is in the main profoundly rational—by far the majority of the text—there is also some explicit recognition of the part played in disease by psychic, divine or demonic influences and past lives and this may be reflected in treatments. In Vimānasthāna VI, passage 3, diseases are classified as curable–incurable, mild or strong, endogenous or exogenous, mental or physical.[81] Elsewhere, exogenous causes include demonic and divine influences.[82] Chattopadhyaya has argued that such passages reflect the fact that the rationalists had bowed to pressure from powerful religious influences to set their work within a religious context.[83] While this may be true, it may also be that the physicians simply recognised some spheres of life that are not completely reducible to material factors and that recognition of such non-physical influences allowed them to address these aspects of a patient's understanding and bring this within their purview, hence maintaining their position.

---

79. Ibid., 405.
80. Ibid., 100.
81. Ibid., 183.
82. Ibid., vol. I 159, Sūtrasthāna VII 51-52. For disease due to vitiation of mind, emotions, senses or psyche see Sūtrasthāna VIII 15, vol. I 169-170; Vimānasthāna VI, 8 vol. II, 187. For divine or demonic influences, see Vimānasthāna III 19-20, vol. II 147; Sūtrasthāna XX 4, vol. I, 360, Śārīrasthāna VI 27, vol. II 445; Vimānasthāna III 22-23 and 29-37, vol. II 148-149 and 151-155; Nidānasthāna I 35, vol. II 29.
83. Chattopadhyaya (1979) Chapter 2.

Knowing a person's *prakṛti* is vital for the physician (Śārīrasthāna VI, passage 3; Vimānasthāna VIII, 94).[84] The basic constitutional types or *prakṛtis* are those dominated by a particular *doṣa*. Thus we have *vata*, *pitta*, or *kapha* types of patients. In some types there is an even balance among the three *doṣas* (Vimānasthāna VIII, passage 100 and Sūtrasthāna VII, verses 39-40).[85]

## Therapeutic Strategies in *Caraka*

Treatment for imbalanced *doṣas* is by a variety of means including:

- diet and exercise regimens (Sūtrasthāna V, VI, VII, 31-35, XXVII, XXVIII (34-42); further examples are found in Cikitsāsthāna).
- drugs and treatments which promote first the detachment and removal of a deranged *doṣa* from its abnormal site and then elimination of its excess from the body through the excretory channels (bowels, urine, skin), the mouth or nasal orifices by means of medicated enemas (*basti*), emetics (*vamana*) and nasal applications (*nasya*) (Sūtrasthāna I, 80-92; IV entire chapter ; Vimānasthāna, VIII 150-151; Cikitsāsthāna III, 146-177).
- drugs and foods to strengthen a diminished doṣa; depending on their tastes and qualities, e.g. light or heavy (Sūtrasthāna XXVI,11-36; XXVII entire chapter).
- fomentations and sweat baths (*sveda*), massage with oils and ingestion of oils (*sneha*) (Sūtrasthāna chapters XIII and XIV).
- blood letting and cautery (Cikitsāsthāna V, 32,60-64; IX,70).

Together these make-up *pañcakarma* or the five therapeutic actions: emesis, enema, purgation, nasal cleansing, and blood purification by letting.

Two basic approaches to treatment are lightening (*laṅghana*) and increasing (*bṛhmana*) (Sūtrasthāna XXII). One of these is chosen as the main approach. A third type of treatment,

84. Sharma and Dash vol. II 426; 261-266.
85. Ibid., 267 and vol. I 154.

*rasāyana*, is to strengthen and improve overall vitality in the patient once he or she has recovered. It is also given in the healthy individual for maintenance (Cikitsāsthāna I, parts 14). A fourth type, *vājīkaraṇa*, aims to maintain sexual potency as an indicator of overall vitality (Cikitsāsthāna II, parts 1-4). The basic principles behind these treatments are the association of like to like and the antagonism of opposites to balance the individual *prakṛti* through foods, drugs, and adjustments to habitation, seasons, time of day, age.

## Vāta and Ojas

Before closing this survey, two more features of the system should be considered. The first is the prominence and overall importance given to the *vāta* humour. That *vāta* is specially important is shown by the extra text given over to its description, as well as to individual statements. Thus one chapter is entitled "The merits and demerits of *Vāta*" (Sūtrasthāna XII); and although it includes a discussion of *pitta* and *kapha*, most of the text discusses *vāta*. In this chapter, *vāta* is described as the bodily aspect of the natural *vayu* or air in the world outside the body. *Vāyu* is said to have the following actions: sustenance of the earth, kindling of fire, bringing about compactness and movement in the sun, moon, stars, planets, creation of clouds, showering of rains, flowing of rivers, bringing about maturity of flowers, and fruits, shooting forth the plants, classification of seasons and the five *mahābhūtas*, manifesting the shape and size of the products of the five *mahābhūtas*, bringing about the power of germination in seeds and growth of plants, bringing about hardness and dryness in the grains and bringing about transformation everywhere.[86]

*Vāyu-vāta's* disruptive activities are also enumerated in this passage: how it can destroy when it is excessive. Vāta is further related to the wind-god *Vāyu*, subtle and omnipresent, permeating the whole universe. While *kapha* is related to *Soma*, god of the moon and waters, much less detail is given and it is not characterised as omnipresent, permeating the whole universe. Finally, the text concludes,

86. Ibid., vol. I 238 Sūtrasthāna XII, 7.

> If a physician does not comprehend the *vāyu* which excels in strength, roughness, quickness and destructive power, how would he be able to forewarn a patient well in advance of its disastrous effects and how would he advise about the normal quaiities of *vāyu* conducive to good health, improvement of strength and complexion, lustre, growth, attainment of knowledge and longevity?[87]

In another part of *Caraka Saṃhitā*, it is stated there are eighty diseases due to *vāta,* while fewer, forty, are caused by *pitta* and twenty by *kapha* (Sūtrasthāna XX, passages 11-19).[88] This also suggests that *vāta* is responsible for or implicated in the greater number of diseases.

Although all three *doṣas,* as representatives of the cosmic elements in the body, are needed for health, *vāta* is seen as particularly important, as its prominence in the text demonstrates. *Vāta* is responsible for movement and for the regularity of that movement, which is essential for health. If *vāta* is disturbed, all other process in the organism are thrown awry. Furthermore, *vāta*'s qualities include coolness and dryness. If these particular aspects of its qualities are increased, the organism can also be particularly threatened. For the Ayurvedic physician, health is equated with equilibrium of *doṣas* and *dhātus.* As we have seen in the discussion of digestion, it is also equated with healthy digestion through *agni,* a function of *pitta.* Finally the normal balance of moisture and fluids in the body—a function of *kapha*—is also important. While any *doṣa* can disturb the other two and thus cause disease processes, a disturbance of *vāta doṣa* creates a more profound imbalance. As the source of movement, when disturbed it can disrupt the normal movement of the other two, or displace them from their normal sites. Being responsible for the movement of wastes out of the body, its blockage can create problems. Its excess can over-heat *pitta* or dry out *kapha.*

The chapter on *vāta* says that it "*consists of prāṇa, udāna, samāna, apāna and vyāna.*"[89] These are the five types of

87. Ibid., 240 Sūtrasthāna XII, 10.
88. Ibid., 363-372.
89. Ibid., 237.

*prāṇa*; although the text does not go on to explain these terms, Filliozat does discuss their meanings. *Vāta,* the air principle, is not seen merely as the *doṣa* of respiration. *Prāṇa* is the breath of the front, of inspiration, the inward moving air. *Udāna* is the breath which goes upwards and makes speech possible. *Samāna* is the concentrated breath of the middle of the body, the air available for maintaining digestive fire (fire needs air). *Apāna* is downward moving breath and motivates the functions of excretion via the urinary tract and bowels and also childbirth. *Vyāna* is the diffused breath which permeates the whole body, making possible the movement of the limbs. In other texts of Ayurveda, five *pittas* and five *kaphas* are also enumerated. These are included in Ayurvedic medicine, but in *Caraka* only *vāta* is singled out for this more detailed refinement and discussion.

In addition, *vāta* is also especially related to the psycho-spiritual aspect of human life. The inclusion of a reference to Vāyu the Vedic god of wind is perhaps significant as it connects the physicians with a more ancient tradition in which vāyu was the divine breath. Filliozat has shown that in the period of the Vedas, Vāyu, the wind god, was identified with the natural wind and with breath. Its action is sometimes assimilated with that of the sun and of fire and is found in the body as breath (*prāṇa*) and soul (*ātman*).[90] From Sāṃkhya philosophy as represented in Chapter I of Śārīrasthāna, we find the concept of the soul (*puruṣa*) as consciousness (verse 16). *Vāta doṣa* as the embodiment of the wind principle is thus particularly important and most specifically related to mind, consciousness and eternal soul.

Similar emphasis on the primacy of wind is found in other ancient texts of Āyurveda, Bheda, and also in Suśruta, though with less emphasis on wind as a cosmic force. Filliozat concludes:

> The three great Indian texts of medicine are thus unanimous in making the wind as the soul of the world and of the body, in the concrete sense of the word 'soul'. The various winds, organic breaths or 'animal spirits' are the principles of the entire manifestation of life in the body.[91]

90. Filliozat (1964) 62-66.
91. Ibid., 218.

The air *doṣa, vāta,* responsible for breath and movement, is the life principle *par excellence* and underpins the other two *doṣas* and their functions in the body. When it is disturbed it is bound to affect the other two. If a disease either begins with a direct disturbance of *vāta,* or progresses from a relatively superficial stage of disturbance of *kapha* or *pitta* to a stage where *vāta* also becomes disturbed, the disease is more life-threatening.

Another vital component of the body is *ojas. Ojas* is a vital fluid constituent. It is closely akin to the *kapha doṣa*; both represent the embodiment of the water as vital element. However, *ojas* is distinct from *kapha.* It is conceived as a more subtle fluid element. It is said to dwell in the heart and to be necessary to the existence of the vital air (*prāṇa*)[92] indicating the mutual need between moisture and air principles. When diminished, its signs and symptoms are

> the fear complex, constant weakness, worry, affliction of sense-organs with pain loss of complexion, cheerlessness, roughness, and emaciation.[93]

These are almost exactly the main symptoms of derangement of the *vāta doṣa,* whose qualities include dryness, roughness, and the emotions of fear and anxiety.

These are some of the main features of the Ayurvedic concept of doṣas in relation to health and disease according to Caraka. As we proceed to examine the related concept of humours in the Hippocratic *Corpus,* we will be able to notice strong similarities.

## CHARACTERISTICS OF THE HIPPOCRATIC HUMOURS

Before looking at the nature of the humours individually, let us consider some of their characteristics as a whole, and how knowledge about humours was put to use in diagnosis and treatment.

---

92. Sharma and Dash vol. I (1994) 595, Sūtrasthāna XXX, 9-11.
93. Ibid., 325, *Sūtrasthāna* XVII, 73-76.

## Coction, Mixture, and Separation

Reflecting the general Greek view that having anything in isolation is threatening to the ideal of balance and harmony, the humours, or in the case of *Ancient Medicine* tastes, are said to be normal and healthy constituents when they are mixed[94] and to become pathological when they become unmixed.[95] Being unmixed allows them to be separated[96] hence too strong,[97] upsetting the balance with their influence. Being well-mixed or compounded [98] allows them to remain mild and healthful (*Ancient Medicine*, XIV, XIX, *Sacred Disease*, XII, XIII). What keeps them mixed is proper coction.[99] In treatment, the aim is to return the humours to normal by coction. Writers sometimes also use the term 'mature' for this return to normalcy. This is closely connected to the idea of coction because fruits and vegetables are said to become mature through the warming power of the sun which in effect 'cooks' them, bringing them to fruition. Again the human body is seen as intimately connected to the same processes that occur in wider nature.

When observing the patient, the physician looks for signs showing lack of coction or presence of coction (maturity) in the humours. An example of a sign of a humour changing from unmixed to mixed and concocted is when urine changes from being thin and/or watery, turbid (having suspended particles in it) or cloudy, 'crude' frothy or black (dark), to being thick (relatively), pure or clear, uniform or smooth, and forming a healthy (white) sediment. Similarly, stools change from being bilious, 'crude', thin-watery, irritating or smarting, or uncompounded to concocted—normal, formed stools. Sweats and the types of sweats were also watched for.

> In all acute diseases those sweats are best that occur on the critical days and completely get rid of the fever. Those too are good that occur all over the body, showing that the

---

94. *memigmena,* Jones (1972) vol. I 38, 42.
95. *akreton,* Ibid., 38.
96. *apokrithe,* Ibid.
97. *ischuron,* Ibid.
98. *kekretai,* Ibid. See also vol. II 165.
99. *pephthenta,* Ibid., 49.

> patient is bearing the disease better. Sweats without one of these characteristics are not beneficial (*Prognostic* VI).[100]

One main aim of a therapy is to bring the deranged humours back to maturity. Coction returns them to the normal consistency; if they are too thin, maturity would show in their thickening; if too thick, in their becoming thinner. *Ancient Medicine* XIX describes discharges: "where acrid and unmixed humours come into play...the cause is the same, and...restoration results from coction and mixture."[101] Once concocted, they are directed out of the body, through stools, urine, sweat or vomiting, with medicines, diet, and exercise. These treatments encourage the body to do what it naturally knows to do. *Ancient Medicine* XIX describes bile leaving the body "when the patient gets rid of it, sometimes by purgation, either spontaneous or by medicine..."[102] In some cases it is only necessary to bring them back to their normal condition and site within the body, i.e. phlegm to its normal proportions, similarly bile and blood. The opening of the treatise on *Humours* states:

> The colour of the humours, where there is no ebb of them, is like that of flowers. They must be drawn along the suitable parts whither they tend, except those whose coctions comes in due time.[103]

Again here we find that the humours are thought to move and to tend to move in certain directions or to certain sites. Such 'drawing' was done in various ways. For example, by stimulating purgation through the 'lower cavity', the bowel (*Epidemics* I, case II) with suppositories or with herbs such as hellebore a humour may be drawn down. By fomentations (hot) to melt the humours they are encouraged to be released through the skin with sweat. Signs of maturity are favourable signs for the outcome:

> In all dangerous cases you should be on the watch for all favourable coctions of the evacuations from all parts or for

100. Jones (1981) vol. II 15.
101. Jones (1972) vol. I 49.
102. Ibid.
103. Jones (1979) vol. IV 63.

fair and critical abcessions.[104] Coctions signify nearness of crisis and sure recovery" (*Epidemics* I, XI)[105]

An example, appears in *Epidemics* III, case III: towards the twentieth day, the fever has stopped, the urine became thin but by the twenty-fourth to seventh days it had sediment; on the fortieth day the patient passed motions full of phlegm, white or rather frequent and had a copious sweat all over, indicating a perfect crisis.

## Flowing, Moving, Melting, Instability and Change

Our etymology of the word humour included the ideas of flowing and melting, which is what fluids are capable of doing. This associated aspect seems important to the Hippocratic concept for the humours. When pathological, humours create fluxes, flow or run down and melt. (*Humours, Airs Waters, Places, Affections, Places in Man*).[106] When a humour becomes separated and thus stronger it also puts itself in motion.[107] It then flows to another part of the body. Humours, as well as being fundamental constituents of the entire body, were also considered to be especially associated with certain sites in the body.[108] The brain, bone marrow and generative organs are the main site of the moisture principle, phlegm. The liver or sometimes simply the area below the diaphragm, including the upper stomach, is the site of bile and also is especially associated with blood. The heart also later comes to be seen as not so much as a main site of blood, but as intimately connected with the healthy flow of blood. Blood was earlier recognised as being in the lungs.[109] Heart and lungs are also particularly associated with air, as vital breath.

---

104. Abcessions are an accumulation of morbid matter in an area of the body prior to its being eliminated. Remaining unconcocted, abcesses can turn bad, denoting an absence of crisis and prolonging of illness.
105. Jones (1972) vol. I 163.
106. *rue, rei* Potter (1995) 36, *suntekontai*, Jones (1972) 84, Potter (1988) 40.
107. *kinesis* Jones (1979) 86.
108. See Onians (1994) 84-85 (bile, liver), 118 (water, brain, spinal fluid/marrow), 121 (seed, sperm) and also Lonie (1981) for his commentary on *Diseases* IV 55 ff.
109. Onians (1994) 47-48.

The spleen is associated with water and yet, at the same time, with melancholy, as will be discussed below.

When not at its normal site, a humour causes pathological changes. A humour in movement becomes a flux.[110] When a humour is set in motion, it can then settle in another part of the body and cause problems. In *Affections* 11 phrenitis is said to "arise from bile which is set in motion and settles in the inward parts and the diaphragm."[111] A humour such as phlegm may flow in extra amounts to the brain, its natural reservoir, causing an excess there. It is then said to condense, putrefy and become noxious. From there it can spread throughout the body by virtue of its naturally heavy nature and gravity.[112]

*Decorum* XIII states, "for instability is characteristic of the humour and so they may be easily altered by nature and by chance." This sentence points out an important characteristic of the humours: their ability to change and transform. They are not static but dynamic, hence the health of the body is also not a state of constant perfection but a dynamic process. Disease too can be 'turned'. This is perhaps not surprising if we remember the humours are above all fluids and thus epitomise transformation from one state to another. Particular humours, while being associated with certain organs or functions in the body, can also cause problems at other sites in the body. At its new site a humour can provoke disease. For example, in *The Sacred Disease,* IX, excess phlegm congested in the brains of infants descends to the heart and lungs, causing palpitation and difficulty breathing, through chilling of the blood. In *Disease IV,* 40.3 a humour in an organ which is not its natural reservoir causes a disease. Also if a condition caused by one humour does not resolve itself, it can involve other humours, or it could be said the humour transforms or alters itself into another humour.[113]

Melting is one way in which both the humours and tissues of the body change. It would seem to carry with it the idea that the

---

110. Thivel (1981) 351.
111. Potter (1988) 21.
112. Thivel (1981) 350-351.
113. *astata, eumetapoenta, phusis, tuches* Jones (1981) vol. II 294, 157-158. Lonie (1981) 27.

humour has lost its proper or normal constituency or integrity, and thus begins to flow out of its proper sphere. This can disrupt the balance of other humours or organs and thus of the body as a whole. (*Places in Man*, 1 points out that disease in one part creates disease in others and that every part communicates with every other.) According to *Airs, Waters and Places*, VII when frosty waters are drunk it is conducive to phlegm and to large stiff spleens along with hard, thin, hot stomachs and emaciation, because the flesh melts or dissolves to feed the spleen. In chapter X inhabitants of a city exposed to hot winds but sheltered from north winds will have heads moist and full of phlegm with digestive organs imbalanced because of the phlegm which has melted and runs down into them from the head. *The Art*, XIV states that heat warmer than the natural heat will melt the 'matters' [humours]. In *Regimen II*, 66, improper exercise can cause overheating which melts the flesh, causing an imbalance of moisture in the body, which collects in a particular place, causing pain. If it becomes fixed there through lack of circulation, it can become too hot and go on to cause fever. In *Diseases IV*, 45, either too much or too little exercise causes melting of a humour which then results in imbalance.[114]

A humour can accumulate to excess in one season, yet not flow from its site or manifest its imbalance until the next. *Nature of Man, VII* explains how the winter

> fills the body with phlegm...the sputum and nasal discharge of men is fullest of phlegm; at this season mostly swellings become white and diseases generally phlegmatic. And in spring too phlegm still remains strong in the body, while the blood increases. For the cold relaxes [with the warmth of spring] and the rains come on, while the blood accordingly increases.[115]

An example of a humour flowing, and spreading to affect other humours and transforming would be the following passage from *Diseases I*, chapter 30:

---

114. Potter (1995) vol. VIII 19; *suntekontai* Jones (1972) vol. I 84-85; 75; (1981) vol. II 217; (1979) vol. IV 359-360; Lonie (1981) 30.
115. Jones (1979) vol. IV 19.

> Phrenitis is as follows: blood contributes the greatest part to his intelligence...therefore when bile that has been set in motion enters the vessels and the blood it stirs the blood up, heats it and turns it to serum, altering its normal consistency and motion.... Patients with phrenitis most resemble melancholics in their derangement, for melancholics too, when their blood is disordered by bile and phlegm, have this disease and are deranged—some even rage. In phrenitis, the raging and derangement are less in the same proportion that this bile is weaker than the other one [i.e. black bile].[116]

However, such states of imbalance or instability are at one and the same time pathological and curative, for the disease manifested is seen as a natural and rational defence reaction of the body, a way of returning itself to its norm, after finding itself in exceptional circumstances.[117]

A corollary of this is that the physician can use medicines, diet, exercise—even the 'therapeutic word'—to support and mimic nature's efforts to re-balance the humours.[118] *The Art* speaks of "nature constrained to give up her secrets" (XIII) and of medicine discovering "drinks and food of such a kind that,

---

116. Potter (1988) vol. VI 177, 179. See also (1995) 43.
117. Jones (1981) vol. II 215 *The Art* XIII.
118. While making use of Lain Entralgo's highlighting of the 'therapeutic word', (Chapter Four) I would disagree with his conclusions that the physicians did not make use of it fully. It is true that there is not much evidence for its use in the *Corpus*. As Lain Entralgo has pointed out there is ample evidence that they certainly recognised the importance of the psychic life in their patients. Yet let us bear in mind that a substantial amount of the treatments in the *Corpus* are dealing with highly acute, often life threatening diseases and fevers, and in such cases reestablishing a physical equilibrium in the body is the first priority. The physicians may have left to temple medicine the treatment of more chronic or psychologically complex afflictions. Also, we do not know for sure that other lost treatises may not have dealt with these matters; those we have are the treatises which have survived because they were most useful for physicians for the diseases they were witnessing. Finally, their emphasis on prognosis, being able to speak to the patient about his disease, and its symptoms that he himself may not have noticed or mentioned, and to foretell accurately the progress of the disease (or its incurability as the case may be) is in part employing the therapeutic word to gain their confidence and put their minds at ease, so that the physical side of treatment could have its fullest effect.

becoming warmer than the natural heat, melt the matters I spoke of and make them flow away, which they never would have done without this treatment."[119] *Regimen I,* XV states "nature knows how to do these things.... In other respects too nature is the same as the physician's art."[120]

*Aphorisms* VII, LIV shows that the physicians knew how to move an imbalanced humour to the right channels that would take it out of the body: "In cases where phlegm is confined between the midriff and stomach, causing pain because it has no outlet into either of the cavities, the disease is removed if the phlegm be diverted by way of the veins into the bladder."[121] Similarly, *Aphorisms* I, XXI states, "What matters ought to be evacuated, evacuate in the direction to which they tend, through the appropriate passages."[122] The idea is to support what the body is observed to do itself in such cases—letting nature be the teacher. Since the body tries to expel imbalanced humours by creating vomit, sweats, and evacuations such as diarrhoea, so the physicians mimic and support this effort with their own treatments, as the passages in *Nature of Man* VI and *The Art* quoted above show(pp. 68, 173). The humour needs to be led out of the body after it has been either concocted, or broken up. The physicians definitely felt they could control the humours through regimen, drugs and external applications, such as vapour baths, oiling, fomentations, cupping, as well as venesection. *Epidemics* 2.3.8 states:

> create apostases, leading the material yourself. Turn aside apostases that have already started, accept them if they come where they should and are of the right kind and quantity, but do not offer assistance. Turn some aside if they are wholly inappropriate, but especially those that are about to commence or are just begun.[123]

*Nature of Man*, V also notes the physician's ability to give a certain drug to evacuate particular humours.

---

119. Jones (1981) vol. II 215.
120. Jones (1979) vol. IV 253, 255.
121. Ibid., 205, 207.
122. Ibid., 107.
123. Smith (1994) vol. VII 57. An apostasis is like an abcession, a deposit or an excretion of diseased matter.

Another aid to the physician's art is the use of the 'therapeutic word'. Part of the declaration of the prognosis was to gain the confidence of the patient. But a more explicit example was cited in Chapter Two: in *Regimen IV,* LXXXIX the physician prescribes laughter therapy as a treatment for anxiety. The patient should "address his mind to theatrical performances, [audio-visual therapeutics] especially those that bring laughter, otherwise those that please him most."[124]

## Excess, Congealing and Gathering

In addition to the imbalance of isolation, humours may also become pathological if they become excessive, if there is a surfeit of the humour.[125] This is another way a humour can become too strong. This can happen both at the natural site of the humour or if it moves to a site which is not its normal one. If there does occur a surfeit or excess of a humour, it is sometimes said to become collected and to block or congeal a body process or part, thus preventing that part from fulfilling its normal healthy function.[126] This is usually the phlegmatic humour for its nature is already to be cool and coldness is associated with congealing. Melancholy too can have a chilling, blocking effect, creating spasms. The hotter or more drying humours, bile or melancholy, and even phlegm when overheated (see p. 184), when excessive or separated assert their negative influence through burning and/or dryness. For anything that suffers either heat or cold too long becomes dry. (Ice is drying and brittle.) In *Regimen II,* LXVI excess moisture tends to gather and causes pain until it passes out, or remaining still grows hot, overpowers the healthy parts and creates a fever in the whole body.[127]

Pneuma can also be harnessed for treatment. Again a passage in *Regimen I,* XXXI states that in the case of a woman who aborts, often the treatment is to insert a pessary into the womb, but also to give a diet to generate the most air possible in the womb. Cupping may have been thought to work via pneuma.[128]

---

124. Lain Entralgo's translation (1970 163).
125. *plesmone* Jones (1979) vol. IV 384-385.
126. *sunestekos* Ibid., 360-361, *pexai* Jones (1981) vol. II 164.
127. *sunsistatai* Ibid., 358.
128. Jones (1979) vol. IV 273; Lonie (1981) 268. Contemporary herbalists also use herbal pessaries to heal locally in the vagina and womb.

## Constitution, Nature and Prognosis

If man is constituted of certain humours, individual men are constituted of varying proportions of each of these constituents. The proportion of the humours in a person define that individual's *katastasis* or constitution, his inherent nature or individual *phusis*. His physique may also be related to the predominance of a particular humour in his make up. If phlegm is the predominant humour, he is said to be phlegmatic, if bile is strong, bilious, etc. These constitutions or natures are constantly related to the other aspects of human experience; to foods (*Ancient Medicine, Regimen* I), to exercise (*Regimen in Acute Diseases, Regimen* II), to climate, setting of habitation, drinking waters and seasons (*Airs Waters, Places, Humours* XII, *Aphorisms* III, XVI, *Regimen II, Epidemics* 4, 46) to the times of day (*Epidemics*, 6.1,11), and stages of life (*Regimen in Health*, II; *Humours* XVI, *Nature of Man*, VII, XV, *Regimen I*, XXXII).

From the physician's point of view, a person's constitution has important implications for his health and knowing a person's inherent nature, as well as being able to recognise it along with the nature of the disease, helps the physician understand how the patient becomes ill and how to treat his illness. The disease also is sometimes spoken of as having a nature of its own: it is a bilious, phlegmatic, sanguine or melancholic disease. *Humours* XIII says that physicians need to be able to foretell what the "character of a season's diseases and constitutions will be...."[129] *The Sacred Disease* attributes epilepsy ultimately to a combination of pneuma and phlegm, the phlegm blocking the proper flow of pneuma. It is a phlegmatic disease.

*Prognostic* states: "It is necessary to learn the natures of such diseases, how they exceed the strength of men's bodies and to learn how to forecast them." For the physician, a disease of a certain nature will be expected to display certain types or qualities of symptoms which correspond to those of that humour. Knowing a patient's inherent balance of humours helps the physician understand how he will react to his surroundings, environment,

129. Jones (1979) vol. IV 85.

food and to any pathological processes set in motion within him. *Epidemics* 2, 8 states:

> The original nature is the effective thing. One must consider also what comes from way of life...For each thing consider what its growth reduces and what its reduction increases; for the increases what kinds of things are increased with them and what kinds are suppressed.

We have also seen an example of this in the passage quoted above from *Diseases I,* 30 where the naturally melancholic constitution with phrenitis would still have less bile and therefore rage less. *Aphorisms* II, XVII the amount of nourishment must be compatible with the constitution, or disease is caused. This reminds the physician to take account of the patient's constitution or nature when prescribing both curative and health maintaining treatments. Also if the nature of the disease is like that of the patient, the season, his age and habits, it is less dangerous for him than when there is no relationship (*Aphorisms* II, XXXIV).[130]

Such observations and discernments are essential to the physician in using his medical reasoning. as we have seen above. *Epidemics* I, XI states: "Declare the past, diagnose the present, foretell the future."[131] The physician needs to understand how a particular disease occurred in a particular patient, how it is manifested in the present and how it will behave in the future. These things should be communicated to the patient and his co-operation enlisted in overcoming the disease.

## Therapeutic Methods

Knowing both the nature of the patient, the nature of the season and the nature of his disease, also helps the physician choose the appropriate therapy. *Humours* XII sums it up: "some [diseases] are the result of the physical constitution, others of regimen, of the constitution of the disease, of the seasons." When the affections do not accord with the patient's nature, the physician

130. Jones (1981) vol. II 7-9; Smith (1994) vol. VII 27; Potter (1988) vol. V 179; Jones (1979) vol. IV 117.
131. Jones (1972) vol. I 165.

must examine the circumstances and the signs and symptoms of the patient, according to *Epidemics* 2.3. In particular he must note what increases or reduces each factor. (*Epidemics* 2.1.8)[132]

Knowing these factors, treatments would be often by opposites, as we have seen in the breaking up congested humours. *Aphorisms* II, XXII states," Diseases caused by repletion are cured by depletion...in general contraries are cured by contraries." In another example, a treatment for a spasm, [a cold affliction] is to give warmth. (*Epidemics* 2.5,21) The treatment strategy could also be to encourage the augmentation of a particular humour by administering like substances, based on the idea that likes attract likes; for example one who is cool, thin and weak would be given foods or medicaments that encourage digestion and build tissue: foods like olive oil that are fat, rich and sweet promote moistness, phlegm and strength (*Affections* 55).[133]

Treatment methods included: herbs, taken internally and applied externally in poultices and vapour baths, different types of healing diets or fasts, exercises, both wet and dry fomentations with salt or toasted millet, baths and massages. For example, the aim of treatment for congested or congealed humours was to break them up, especially by the use of vapour baths or fomentations. The treatment in *Regimen II,* LXVI above is by means of vapour baths and hot baths, exercise and diet to "break up the collected humour", followed by oiling the body. This is a form of sweating therapy with the use of aromatic herbs. This is a common treatment found in the *Corpus* and usually orthodox scholars have considered it either of no affect or part of the mild and gentle methods of the Hippocratic physicians, which could only be slightly effective, if at all. However, the practice is still used by naturopathic and herbal practitioners to release build-up of toxins through the skin. Furthermore, contemporary research and developments in the field of essential oil therapy have amply proved that essential oils are absorbed through the skin and lungs, go directly into the blood stream and from there

132. Jones (1979) vol. IV 85; Smith (1994) vol. VII 27.
133. Ibid., 113; Smith (1994) vol. VII, 79; Potter (1988) vol. V, 85.

throughout the body, being particularly excreted through the breath and urine. These essential oils and the herbs from which they derive—the form in which the Greek physicians would have used them—are now known to have diaphoretic, anti-bacterial and anti-viral effects. One of the classic treatment methods of Āyurveda is the sweating or *svedana* with aromatic herbs simmering to create the steam, followed by oiling, a therapeutic practice which is still being used clinically in Ayurvedic hospitals in India today.

A person's nature or constitution was not just confined to aspects of the physical body but also included the mental- emotional aspects. As will be discussed more fully below, each humour had certain corresponding characteristic mental-emotional dispositions associated with it.

Physicians also considered the mental–emotional aspect of the patient in their treatments. *Epidemics* 2.4 states "it is appropriate to induce anger for the sake of restoring colour and humours, also to induce happiness, fear and the like. If the rest of the body is ill it should be treated at the same time. Otherwise just this."[134] In other words, some imbalances in humours would affect just the mental-emotional sphere and could be treated on that level.

The most discussed constitutions in the treatises are those of bile and phlegm. In *Nature of Man* and *Diseases IV* are added two more humours and two more constitutional types, sanguine/blood and melancholy/black bile in the case of *Nature of Man*, and sanguine/blood and water/splenetic in the case of *Diseases IV*. Apart from their appearance in these more 'theoretical' treatises, bilious, sanguine, phlegmatic and melancholic constitutions are also recognised in the practical ones, for example, *Regimen I, II, III*; *Epidemics* I, 2.3,5; 4,28.

## Characteristics of the Individual Humours

*Phlegm*: In the treatises, phlegm is the humour associated with coldness and moisture, but also with fevers. It is mentioned as a

134. Smith (1994) vol. VII 73.

contributory cause in epilepsy, in catarrhs and as appearing in vomits. Observation and medical reasoning taught the physicians that phlegm and what it represents, moisture and coolness, was necessary to the body to maintain a certain degree of coolness to balance innate heat. Moisture was also necessary to life,[135] but if it became excessively increased, imbalance occured and hence disease. Phlegm was more evident in the damp, cold of winter, and hence people with phlegmatic constitutions suffer more from phlegm in winter. Another practical observation concerned the material of the brain (viewed in butchered animals, in wounds to the head which exposed its contents). This material was pale and wet. In non-medical literature it was related to the soul.[136] We do find in the *Corpus* that phlegmatic diseases very often are caused by imbalance in which phlegm runs down from the head and causes disturbance to the rest of the body. The head or brain with its cerebral marrow is like a reservoir of the phlegm, which is also present throughout the body. *Fleshes* states "the brain is the metropolis of the cold and gluey."[137] This cerebral-spinal marrow, being a fluid, is for the Greeks a vital sap and equated with life and procreation.[138] In *On Generation* we find the idea that the seed enters the spinal marrow and from there travels through vessels (these may not necessarily be the physical vessels in the body) to the kidneys and beyond to the testes and penis. Women, too, are thought to have a natural vital fluid in their reproductive organs. When the seed of man and woman are united in intercourse, a child is conceived. Interestingly, the man's fluid is thought to be cooler than the woman's, although

135. Onians (1994) 289, 272-274.
136. Ibid., 120, n. 4.
137. The description is also found in Aristotle's *de Part. Anim.* 652a, 21, as Onians points out, ibid.
138. Ibid., 221- 229. Onians points out, p. 210, that this also explains the practice of anointing, and the application of oily liquids after the bath—they "introduce into the body through the pores, the stuff of life and strength." Hence for the physician, the use of massage with oily liquid would have been a means of restoring vitality to the body.

otherwise men are thought naturally warmer than women in nature or constitution.[139]

Phlegm is thus the principle of moisture and coolness, the cosmic water element represented in the body. Yet etymologically, *phlegma* is associated with heat, and in the treatises phlegm is seen as responsible for heat, swellings and inflammations and sometimes fevers. This at first seems inconsistent. Logically, would not excessive cold create an imbalance of cold symptoms rather than of hot ones? Following Jouanna, Thivel has suggested that phlegm, while not hot in itself, causes heat by its reactions and that this exemplifies the play of concepts of similars and opposites.[140] The physicians reasoned that phlegm, though cold, produces inflammation when it 'bears' the fleshes, that which it must not do. It is the operation of the principle of contraries, cold produces heat. Thivel concludes that "for the ancients, the humour in question is not separable from the effect it produces and the same word is used for both."[141] Onians, too, considered this association. He wondered whether the association of phlegm with the brain, in other contexts than the medical, may not also have to do with the belief that the element in the head flamed.[142] In *Ancient Medicine,* XVIII, XIX, as a nasal discharge, phlegm is also sometimes referred to as an acrid humour—acrid suggesting pungent, potentially corrosive, therefore heating. It may also have been based on the observation that in fevers, phlegm is often a factor, often vomited. Here again we have the practical, empirical observations of the physicians. They observe that excess accumulations of an otherwise normal and relatively cool, moist bodily fluid actually provoke heat reactions in the body, or can be determining factors in a feverish disease process.

This practical experience perhaps led them to see a principle of inclusion. Heat and cold are not seen as mutually exclusive or

---

139. Lonie (1981) 1-5 and in *Hippocratic Writings* (Lloyd 1986) 318.
140. Thivel (1981) 349.
141. Thivel (1981) 77-78.
142. Onians (1994) 160, n. 4.

fundamentally separate from each other. Each contains the other, at least potentially. The human body contains moisture, the cooling water element, and also heat as the enlivening innate heat. *Regimen I*, IV :

> Fire has the hot and the dry, water the cold and the moist. Mutually too fire has the moist from water for fire there is moisture and water has the dry from fire, for there is dryness in water also.[143]

Thus, each element or humour has the potential of the other latent within it, a potential which becomes manifest only when an inherent natural balance is disturbed and provokes its appearance.

Phlegm is associated with the season that is predominantly cool and damp, winter (*Nature of Man* VII). Interestingly it was observed that sometimes symptoms of imbalance of phlegm would appear in the following season, spring. Phlegm was also associated with childhood, the body then being more moist. (*Nature of Man* VII, *Aphorisms* III, *Nature of the Child*).

Phlegm is looked for in the urine to determine the state of the disease. If it is congealed, it appears a sediment. If acted on by heat, as in fever, it undergoes coction and can form urinary stones (*Airs, Waters, Places*, IX).

Thivel has postulated that phlegm was seen either as producing a swelling, or as concentrated, which produced inflammation.[144] The author of *Internal Affections* distinguishes between two types of phlegm: a common variety, lasting a short time and easily cured, and a more chronic type. A swelling or abcess (a contained internal swelling) is a sign of the presence of an imbalanced humour which took itself there wrongfully, Thivel points out. The treatment for abcess is cleansing the bowels with herbs, a special diet and exercise regime. Cupping and blood letting are used in prolonged cases.[145]

*Bile:* Bile was understood to be a secretion of the liver, the large blood-gland in the body. Smith states that bile is nowhere

143. Jones (1979) vol. IV 231.
144. Thivel (1981) 306.
145. Potter (1988) vol. VI 137-145.

recognised as part of digestion.[146] Yet he may not be considering the association of the liver and bile with heat and therefore coction, i.e. digestion. Moreover bilious complaints very typically affect the digestion, causing such symptoms as vomiting, a full feeling, burning in the region of the stomach/hypochondria or diarrhoea/dysentery.

Although a bodily fluid, bile, in relation to phlegm, is drier and hotter, and thus also potentially harder. The bilious are said to have "dry ophthalmia because of the warm dryness of their flesh." Bile is also associated with bitterness and the colour yellow. *Ancient Medicine* speaks of an outpouring of the "bitter principle, which we call yellow bile, great nausea, burning and weakness" (XIX).[147] Seasonally, while blood is associated with spring, bile is associated with summer. *Nature of Man*, VII states, "it is chiefly in spring and summer that men are attacked by dysentery and haemorrhaging from the nose, and they are the hottest and red. In summer blood is still strong and bile rises in the body...[in winter] bile being chilled becomes small in quantity". Bile also has a light quality compared to phlegm which is heavy (*Diseases IV*, 36, 1). It is also associated with oiliness, as it arises from oily substances (*Diseases IV*, 49, 3-4 and *Epidemics* 6.5.8).[148]

In pathologies, bile is most associated with the acute fevers and with the blood, for example, *Nature of Man*, XV attributes most fevers to bile, while *Diseases I*, 30 observes that bile that has been set in motion enters the blood, stirs it up and heats it. Fevers are often accompanied by diarrhoea or dysentery, as in 'bilious stools'. Bile can also make the stools hard if its heat dries out the moisture.[149]

Bile is associated with fierceness or acuteness, and with violence. Sacred Disease associates bile and bilious constitutions with violent expressions when it states: "those maddened through bile are noisy, evil-doers and restless, always doing something inopportunate" (XVIII).[150] Anger is the emotion most

146. Smith (1990) 25.
147. Jones (1972) vol. I 49-51.
148. Jones (1979) vol. IV 21; Lonie (1981) 3-4; Smith (1994) vol. VII 257.
149. Ibid., 39; Potter (1988) vol. V 177-179.
150. Jones (1981) vol. II 175.

typical of bile. The Greek term is *cholos* as distinct from *chole*, bile itself, but the closeness is evident. The verb *cholon* means to stir one's bile, or gall and to make angry, embitter. In *Epidemics* 6.5.5 we find that anger, an emotion associated with the liver and bile, "contracts [hardens] the heart and the lungs and draws the hot and moist substances into the head."[151] Onians has shown that this thought is also an expression of general popular thought: *cholos* from the liver is associated with painful emotions, indeed the liver is the "inmost spring of deeper emotions, stirred only by powerful stimuli"; and bile was believed to enter into the organs above the diaphragm, the heart and lungs, as a liquid.[152]

The bilious constitutional type is therefore seen to be more prone to excess of bile, heat and angry emotions. This can be increased or decreased by mode of life, diet, climate or exposure to painful, hurtful emotions. For example, in *Regimen in Acute Diseases*, XXXIV, we read that the bilious, compared to the phlegmatic, does not bear fasting well, and that the naturally bilious are injured by bitter water (LXII).[153]

Treatment for excess bile, as in fevers generally, consists of cooling, moistening foods and herbs and the right type of exercise. When the excess bile has been concocted from a raw to a healthful state, it can be helped out of the body by purging.

*Blood*: This humour is singled out only in a few treatises, though as an important tissue it is often mentioned and can be the focus or cause of disease when acted on by other humours.[154] *Nature of Man* makes it one of the cardinal humours and associates it with spring. It has spring's qualities of moisture and warmth, the qualities of life itself, which return with spring after the death of winter. Blood is also associated with the heart. In *Diseases IV* the heart is the reservoir of blood. As

151. Smith (1994) vol. VII 257.
152. Onians (1994) 85
153. Jones (1981) vol. II 91, 119
154. Lonie (1981) 293. He feels "we have to make a distinction between blood as one of the constituent humours which are the basis of health and disease, and blood as the carrier of life, vitality and in some cases, consciousness. It is the same fluid in each case, but the two uses are very different and sometimes appear contradictory."

the heart-lung area is seen to be easily invaded by the bile from the liver and gall bladder, the blood is particularly susceptible to influence from bile. Yet the liver itself was also known as a large blood gland, so bile's close influence on blood could derive from this view as well.[155] Phlegm can injure blood by chilling or contracting it; air can also.

An earlier treatise, *Airs, Waters, Places,* describes the qualities of spring thus: habitations facing the east, the rising sun, are

> likely to be healthier [because] heat and cold are more moderate...waters are clear, sweet-smelling, soft and delightful... inhabitants are of better complexion, more blooming than elsewhere...A city so situated is just like spring, because the heat and the cold are tempered; the diseases are both fewer and less severe.[156]

In chapter XII we read of a city in Asia Minor, a region "both in character and in the mildness of its seasons,...bearing a close resemblance to spring." As blood comes to be seen as the humour associated with spring, it has these qualities of warmth and temperance between extremes of the heat of summer and the cold of winter.

Although the author of *Nature of Man* gives no great detail about the sanguine constitution or nature, he was not alone in recognising it as a distinct type. *Epidemics* III, 2.15 states: "I think the sanguine and bilious tend to acid belchings and perhaps for those patients it ends in black bile".[157] From its association of blood with the qualities of spring (*Nature of Man* VII) and from the information about spring, we see why *Airs, Waters, Places* shows that the sanguine type will have a typically warm and sunny nature and will be liable to be imbalanced both by the extra heat of bile, acidity or hot, dry weather (summer) and the extra cold, phlegm of winter. The last phrase from *Epidemics* suggests that if the acidity is prolonged, the condition will change to one of black bile. This seems to echo the aetiology of disease in *Nature of Man* as prolonged heat would dry blood's natural moisture, producing melancholy.

---

155. Onians (1994) 47-49, 85; Lonie (1981) 293-294
156. Jones (1972) vol. I 81.
157. Smith (1994) vol. VII 61.

We can get an idea of the physician's concepts about blood as a factor in disease from *Breaths* and *The Sacred Disease* where although not named explicitly as a humour itself, it is the focus of the disease processes in epilepsy. Here blood is changed to a pathological state by the actions of air and phlegm. It is either chilled or compressed by them, both being a form of drying out. Then it begins to disrupt the bodily balance. We have also seen how blood can become toxic from *perissomata* of poor food/ digestion. It can also be 'injured' by bile which over heats, or 'corrupts' it. Such over-heating is most typically seen in fevers.

> The blood heats all the rest of the body and the person, because of the magnitude of his fever and because his blood has become serous and abnormal in its motion, loses his wits and is no longer himself (*Diseases I,* 30).[158]

The physicians found several means of treating blood imbalance. It can be improved by dealing with the humours which may have imbalanced it, e.g. bile or phlegm, or by treating pneuma. By giving herbs to induce vomiting of excess bile, or by a regimen which reduced the excess of bile, phlegm, or air, these humours or factors were restored to normal. Physicians could also act on blood more directly. Having observed that in many fevers there was improvement after spontaneous bleeding from the nose, they sought to imitate this self-healing mechanism by venesection: deliberately bleeding to release the excessive or corrupted blood. Another means of releasing corrupted blood was to bring it to the surface by cupping. From there it could be better released through the superficial levels of the body, the skin. It could also be purged by cleansing the digestive tract with laxative herbs, purging downwards.

*Water*: As a humour water is a prominent feature of *Diseases IV*, which, like *Nature of Man*, views health and disease as a balance between four humours, the fourth in this case being water, rather than melancholy. In this model, instead of relating the humours to seasons, their relation to specific organ sites as

158. Potter (1988) vol. V 179.

'reservoirs' or 'sources' is explicit and the main focus of the aetiology. The water humour is associated with the spleen. The humour is not water *per se* but the watery fluid in the body.[159]

According to *Ancient Medicine,* XXII, and *Diseases IV,* 40.3, the spleen is already a very fluid-filled organ, porous and spongy. To have more water attracted to it causes it to engorge further and, though normally soft and mild, it becomes hard and swollen, since it has no mechanism for either digesting the fluid or evacuating it, as does the bowel with its fluid contents.

The disease most closely associated with such an engorged spleen is dropsy, or swelling, either local or general, in the body.[160] However, in some treatises, there are descriptions of spleen disease which cause emaciation or drying out of flesh. For example, in *Internal Affections,* 33, the spleen becomes engorged with phlegm (another watery humour) and since this prevents the patient from eating properly, he becomes lean and weak. The thinking behind this may be explained by *Airs, Waters, Places,* VII where the spleen of those who drink marshy water enlarges while their stomachs become hard, thin and hot, and their shoulders, collar-bones and faces emaciated. "The fact is that their flesh dissolves to feed the spleen so that they are lean."[161] It is also observed that if water concentrates in the spleen the vital moisture of the body is drawn out of its other tissues, and digestion is prevented. Loss of food emaciates the body. Dryness and emaciation are also a possible effect of melancholy. In *Internal Affections,* 34, the spleen is affected by dark bile in autumn and from the patient drinking water and eating raw vegetables. He again becomes emaciated. *Aphorisms* III, 22 associates enlarged spleen [which accompanies quartan fevers], dropsical and melancholic cases with autumn. According to this evidence, even when water is a cardinal humour, its excessive concentration in one part of the body can bring on the symptoms of melancholy, i.e. drying out of vital moisture and consequent emaciation. In effect these two humours, water and melancholy, are two sides of the same coin.

159. Lonie (1981) 291.
160. Ibid., 292 details the occurrences of this phenomenon in the *Corpus.*
161. Jones (1972) vol. I 85.

The treatment for the watery diseases, such as dropsy, is generally a drying regimen (acid, salty and sour foods) and spleen strengthening herbs. Cautery on the spleen itself was also done. *Internal Affections,* 30 and 31 describes the range of treatments. If the condition has started with watery swelling, but become emaciating at the same time, a balance would be struck between purging the waters and nourishing the body with appropriate diet and rest.

*Melancholy or black bile*: This humour appears in relatively few of the treatises and thus there is less textual evidence than with the other humours to help our understanding. Thivel and Lonie point out that its inclusion as one of four cardinal humours could only occur after Empedocles. According to Thivel, this inclusion was a way the physicians adjusted their model to take account of the newer discoveries of the Italian school of nature philosophers: the roundness of the earth by Parmenides, the harmonics of Pythagoras, the realisation of the heart as the centre of circulation and the "materialising of air" by Empedocles.[162]

The exact nature of black bile is not absolutely clear, although "for over two thousand years it was to play an extremely important part in people's thinking, and not only in medicine."[163] As a humour, to a certain extent it is often evidently just a specific form of bile, yet it was certainly more special than bile's other forms, yellow or acrid, for it was sometimes spoken of as a disease condition in itself. In the treatises melancholy is characterised by a variety of symptoms, mainly loss of normal movement or sensations as in spasms, restlessness, vertigo, with emaciation and weakness, cold and dryness, and with mental derangement. In *Diseases II,* 6 a patient becomes paralysed and speechless when dark bile is set in motion in his head and flows to the chest and cools the blood in other parts causing paralysis. Case 73 describes a patient who vomits up dark material, has variable eating, is unable to see and who wastes away. In case 74 a patient becomes reddish, lean, thin skinned and weak. In *Diseases I,* 3 a patient becomes paralysed as a result of dark bile. In other

162. Thivel (1981) 313.
163. Sigerist (1987) 320.

treatises too, black bile is usually associated with either a physical or mental state of extremity:

*Epidemics* 6, 6.14: a bilious or sanguinous body is melancholic when it lacks evacuation.

*Appendix to Regimen in Acute* 7: several symptoms relating to the nervous system and consciousness are due to flow of dark bile: sensory problems (vision), convulsions, heavy head, epilepsy. Dark bile corrupts the blood, and blocks circulation of air.

*Aphorisms* VI, XVIII: fear or depression *that is prolonged* [emphasis mine], means melancholia.

*Aphorisms* IV, XXIII: it is warned that if black bile be evacuated at the beginning of any disease, whether vomited or purged, it is a mortal sign.[164]

We have seen that warmth and moisture are necessary to the life of the body; however, they must mingle to some degree with their opposites, to keep them wholesome, balanced, to prevent excess. (For separation of any thing, whether it be element, humour, food, or quality, provokes disease.) So the reasoning could have been that there is a place in the body for a healthy proportion of the qualities of dryness and coldness, the qualities of melancholy. It is only when these qualities exceed their healthy proportions that they cause disease.

Jones, examining the possibility that the fevers described in the treatises were in fact various forms of malaria, thought the Greeks observed that protracted malaria (quartan fever which was also attributed to black bile) directly or indirectly produced physical debility and changes of character similar to that also described as melancholia, and thus malaria/black bile could have been one main cause of such symptoms.[165] He notes that in popular speech its meaning approximates to 'nervous breakdown', and included physical and mental prostration.[166] Jones notes

---

164. Smith (1994) vol. VII 267; Potter (1988) vol. VI 269; Jones (1979) vol. IV 185, 129-131, 141.
165. Jones (1909) 96-101.
166. Jones (1972) vol. I lviii, and see (1909) note 6 referring to Aristotles's *Ethics* 1150b on popularity.

that malaria became endemic only in the fifth century and that there is a connection in the medical writings between melancholy, autumn and symptoms of fevers we would call malarial. If so this may help to explain why as a cardinal humour, melancholy makes a later appearance. Again the reasoning would have been based on practical experience and observation.

Sigerist has suggested that, as in other cases, the Greeks based the concept on actual observations. Even today, for example, the stool of patients with bleeding gastric ulcers is black, as is the vomit of patients with stomach carcinoma; a form of malaria produces very dark urine as a result of vascular haemolysis. Similar conditions could have been observed then.[167]

Recently the issue of melanchole has been revisited by P. Voswinckel who presents some overlooked empirical aspects to help explain its existence based on the work of Swedish pathologist Robin Fahraeus (1888-1968). According to Voswinckel, Fahraeus's work shows how blood left to stand in a beaker separates into four layers—a red layer (blood-with oxygen), a whitish layer (fibrin), a yellow layer (serum), and a dark bottom layer. This led him to the conclusion that

> the origin of ancient theory of the four humors and the resulting pathology could only have been understood by the immediate sensory impression of the blood separation.[168]

An excess of this dark bottom layer is associated with certain pathologies: hemoglobinuria, melanogenuria, alkaptonuria, porphrinuria and myglobinuria.[169] At least one of these, porphrinuria, is associated with psycho-mental alterations.

While the above evidence does not entirely clear up the question of what the ancients were witnessing, it at least establishes that they did not simply invent the concept of melancholy to fit pre-existing theoretical assumptions. In addition, it was not only physicians who knew of such conditions: it seems to have existed in popular consciousness long before its appearance in

167. Sigerist (1987) 320.
168. Voswinckel (1990) 1280.
169. Ibid., 1277.

the Hippocratic treatises and had long a history of association with mental states previous to its mention in medical treatises. Jones believes that the fact that melancholia became a popular word shows it was a common occurrence. Both Thivel and Sigerist draw attention to the work of W. Muri. Muri studied this point and found melancholy in many pre-Aristotelian works (such as those of Plato, Aristophanes) and in Menander.[170] In these passages it was seen as the cause of what we would term nervous disturbances such as headache, vertigo, paralysis, spasms, epilepsy as well as serious diseases of quartan fever, and of the kidney, spleen and liver.[171] The term *melagcholan*, according to Muri, meant 'to suffer from the black bile' and must have been commonly used in Attica in the sense of 'to be crazy'.[172] In such passages it seems to be understood as a special form of the bile humour. In the medical writers, Muri found evidence in *Epidemics* I, and 2 to see black bile as a special form of bile, distinguished from its other forms, yellow, red, livid. But in others he finds it as a specific for mental disease because it is present in symptoms of vertigo, troubles with speech and vision, epilepsy, depression with alternating of agitation and langour. Muri finds in these passages the origin of Theophrastus' melancholic character type as recorded in the psuedo-Aristotelian *Problema.*[173] This was the melancholic nature: one characterised by less stability of bodily and mental functions, by irregularity as seen in the fluctuations between states of intense energy and of lethargy, by mental and bodily fluidity or creativity, and those of depletion, depression, spasms, or fear; by a tendency to dryness, slenderness. In extreme cases it was responsible for thinness or emaciation.

Melancholy is quite often not a disease in itself, but appears as a later stage of other diseases, particularly feverish (originally bile or phlegm based) diseases: there is delirium, restlessness and/or lethargy, vertigo or headaches.[174] It is seen as a

170. Sigerist (1961) 320, Thivel (1981) 312.
171. Ibid.
172. Sigerist (1961) 333 n.8.
173. Thivel (1981) 324.
174. See for example: *Diseases I*, 30 (vol. V 179), *Epidemics* III, Case II (vol.I, 261-263).

development of bilious affections.[175] That it can appear as any disease worsens, as if it is the last stage of a condition that may have started by being caused by another humour, is seen by the passage in *Nature of Man*, VI: "But when a man has drunk a drug which withdraws bile, he first vomits bile, then phlegm also. Afterwards under *stress* [emphasis mine] men vomit after these black bile and finally they vomit also pure blood. The same experiences happen to those who drink drugs which withdraw phlegm. First they vomit phlegm, then yellow bile, then black and finally pure blood, whereupon they die."[176] This ability of the humour to appear from a worsening of a disease caused by another humour conforms to the observation discussed above that humours can change from one part of the body to another. Likewise, the disease can change from involving the form of one humour to that of another, as other aspects of the body are compromised. This may also explain how melancholy can develop out of dropsy or engorged spleen, as discussed above. In all these cases it is an extreme state: the body is losing vital moisture, or the proper flow or constitution of water in the body is imbalanced, or the person's ability to move normally is changed (spasms, restlessness with delirium, paralysis), or the senses are affected or there are deranged mental states.

*Epidemics* 6.8.13 states that melancholics become epileptics and epileptics melancholic.[177] Each of these develops more according to what the weakness inclines to more: If the body, epilepsy, if the mind melancholy. This passage affirms that some people may have a constitutional predisposition to one of these two extreme mental states; the same imbalance of humours will affect such people differently. It also suggests that melancholy is more associated with the mental state of the person.

---

175. An interesting light on this progression is the contemporary idea that depression is a kind of 'frozen anger'. We noted the association of anger with the liver, so this would make sense: an anger that cannot be expressed or resolved eventually affects the body in other places or at a deeper level, threatening it now with its 'coldness'.

176. Jones (1979) vol. IV 17, 19.

177. Smith (1994) vol. VII 289.

## The Four Humour Model and Vital Air

Calling *melanchole* a humour and one of four cardinal humours making up the human constitution is a distinguishing feature of the treatise *Nature of Man.* Since this four-humour model was taken up by Galen and became the dominant model in Western medicine until overturned during the scientific and industrial revolutions, we may pause to ask why this four-fold model developed out of the earlier bi-polar or tri-polar models. As said above, it may have been largely due to the influence of the thought of Empedocles, who envisioned the world as deriving from four "root" elements. Having four humours became thus the biological counterpart to this model. But there are other multi-humoural models in the treatises. *Diseases IV* is based on bile, phlegm, water and blood; *Fleshes* on a tri-partite division of qualities into dryness from earth, heat from the heavenly aither and moisture from atmospheric air. Why did that which corresponds so closely to Empedocles eventually become the defining model?

In *Nature of Man,* melancholy is associated with the qualities cold and dry, with the season autumn, when

> blood is least in man, for autumn is dry and begins from this point to chill him. It is black bile which in autumn is greatest and strongest.[178]

Autumn is the time of year associated with approaching death, due in part to its coldness and the disappearance or drying of the sap from plants.

Blood also makes its appearance in this treatise as a humour, though little specific is said about it as a humour. We have the above sentence, a passage in VII associating the nature of blood to that of spring (both are warm and moist) and a passage on venesection in XI. However, the association of blood with the qualities of spring is telling, since the qualities of air in the body as breath are also warmth and moisture and we know that for many physicians, such as the authors of *Breaths* and *The Sacred Disease,* breath is associated with consciousness and the life principle. In these treatises we also find that bile and phlegm affect

178. Ibid., 21.

the blood and consciousness: bile changes blood by an excess of heat, phlegm threatens blood by an excess of cold. Here in *Nature of Man,* VII, we find that the coolness and dryness of autumn, the season when melancholy is "strongest and greatest", contribute to the cooling and lessening of blood, which if unchanged ultimately causes death.

Such an aetiology does reflect the model of the creation described by Empedocles as deriving from four root elements: earth, water, fire and air. If so, though it is not spelled out in the treatise, each of the humours does represent a mingling of some of the qualities of each element: earth is dry, water moist, fire hot and air cold. Thus phlegm is cold and moist, bile hot and dry, sanguine moist and warm and melancholy dry and cold. How did physicians make the connections between the physical and mental diseases they were called upon to treat and traditional concepts about the consciousness, mind–soul or *psyche*?

Thivel believes that once the idea that the heart is the centre of circulation and that the faculty of thought in man is located in the heart and not in the brain, the physicians had to re-formulate their concept. For if so, madness could no longer be attributed to the imbalances in the brain, the reservoir of phlegm. Mental derangements had to be put in relation to the blood and heart: they could only be caused by a "humour", i.e. a constituent element which mixed with blood, so "conforming to the popular idea, they chose black bile at the same time beginning to make it a specific humour."[179] However, this connection of consciousness with the heart-blood could equally be based on other ancient ideas about the breath–soul as located in the chest, though more specifically in the *thumos* or lungs. It would not have been new.

Other considerations may also have been involved in the account of the four humour model, in particular the seasons. Understanding the influence of the seasons is important to Hippocratic diagnosis and prognosis. We know from works such as *Airs, Waters, Places* that physicians observed the strong relationship between locations, climate and seasons on the

179. Ibid., 313.

diseases men are prone to. In this treatise, certain humoural ailments are definitely associated with certain seasons or with the transitions from one season to another. If excess of phlegm builds up in winter, it is said to melt with the warmth of spring and thus begin to flow, or run, causing problems in a later season. This treatise (chapter X) explicitly names four distinct seasons and discusses the types of conditions found in each, how their variations influence disease, and takes into account constitutional variations. *Humours,* XIII also discusses four seasons in relation to conditions that appear. *Regimen III,* LXVIII states "I divide the year into the four parts most generally recognised—winter, spring, summer, autumn."[180] Muri, notes Sigerist,

> makes the very fine observation that until the middle of the fifth century B.C. the Greeks spoke of three seasons only...from the middle of the century on...autumn was looked upon as a season of its own and it may well be that the separation of black bile from bile in general was a similar process.[181]

Therefore, it seems there came to be a clear acceptance of four regular seasons and empirical experience with disease and imbalance in each of these. Melancholy particularly is associated with autumn and with the changes of seasons. The author of *Nature of Man* may have "needed two pairs of humours with opposite qualities and black bile was better than water."[182] Yet he was not the only physician to make these associations. *Regimen I,* XXXII notes that a constitution blended of the rarest fire and the driest water is dry and cold and unhealthy in autumn and healthy in spring; *Internal Affections* describes a hepatic (feverish) disease arising from black bile which flows to the liver. It is said to attack in the fall and at the year's changes.[183]

This last point is also alluded to in *Regimen I,* XII: "For diseases do not arise among men all at once; they gather themselves

180. Jones (1979) vol. IV 369.
181. Sigerist (1961) 334, n. 13.
182. Ibid.
183. Jones (1979) vol. IV 279. Potter (1988) vol. VI 165-167.

together gradually before appearing with a sudden spring."[184] A specific example appears in *Airs, Waters, Places*, X, which discusses how an unseasonably warm winter, followed by a cold spring, brings on disease in the summer due to influences on the body's fluids. These observations find a parallel in Āyurveda in the concept that a *doṣa* can build up in one season unnoticed because other qualities involved in it prevent its manifesting (Sūtrasthāna VI, 22-26). In northern India there are three distinct seasons: summer, rainy and dry. Each *doṣa* is naturally stronger in a season that has the same qualities as itself, but it does not always cause problems until another season. For example, *kapha* can accumulate in winter, but cold prevents it changing or moving, yet any extra heat will provoke it, so that it too causes problems in the spring, when the warmth liquefies it and it begins to run (Sūtrasthāna 22-26). As with the Ayurvedic tradition, it may well be that the Hippocratic physicians, also seeing man as part of his larger physical context, were led by their reasoning to observe more closely the relationship between man and the seasons. Over time, with the accumulation of more information their observations may have become more alert to the connections between the four definite seasons and the health of their patients. The eventual, later development of a four-fold model was more finely tuned to the climate and seasonal variations of ancient Greece.

Yet another consideration, again based on experience, may have been involved. What other phenomenon in nature and in the body has the quality of movement and dramatic change, hence is also a vital principle of life, and yet also, at least potentially, can be cold and dry and thus also threaten life? Anaximenes had perceived that air is the cosmic equivalent of the life–soul in man, and is the originating substance of the universe, with the implicit assumption that man and the larger cosmos are made of the same material and behave according to similar rules.[185] We know that the soul as breath was also a common concept among the ancient Greeks.

---

184. Jones, ibid., 231.
185. Kirk and Raven (1962) 161-162.

> For the Homeric Greeks the *thumos* is the spirit, the breath that is consciousness, variable, dynamic, coming and going, changing as feelings change, and as we may say, as thought changes. Thought and feeling were scarcely separable then and it is still recognised that thought, even the abstract thought of the philosopher, is affected by breathing.[186]

So there was a long-time association in the Greek mind of air, consciousness, and the origin of all movement of the body, breathing. In *Nature of Man* air as an element of nature could thus have been literally incorporated as the aspects of two humours, blood and melancholy.

In other treatises, air is spoken of separately and not as a humour but still as an important component. In *Nature of the Child, Diseases IV*, chapter 17 the attraction of likes which forms the embryo depends originally on the moving force of pneuma in the respiration of the embryo.[187] *Pneuma* is responsible for growth and movement.

The treatise *Breaths* also links these two thoughts. a universal principle of life and movement, *pneuma*, with an individual human manifestation as breath, intelligence or consciousness and movement. For some physicians then, air was not just one of four root elements but a distinctively powerful phenomenon in itself: necessary to life but also capable of disrupting the bodily humoural balance, as it was capable of violence and destruction in nature at large. According to *Breaths*,

> the bodies of men are nourished by three kinds of nourishment...solid food, drink and wind (*pneuma*). Wind in bodies is called breath (*phusa*), outside bodies it is called air (*aer*). It is the most powerful of all and in all.... Such is the power that it has in these things, but it is invisible to sight, though visible to reason (*logismos*). For what can take place without it? In what is it not present? What does it not accompany? For everything between earth and heaven

186. Onians (1994) 50.
187. See Lonie (1981) 9, and commentary 181-182, 301.

is full of wind...for mortals too this is the cause of life and the cause of disease in the sick (III).[188]

Here, as with our definition of the other humours, air is both a normal healthy presence in the body, symbolic of and necessary even to its life, and at the same time a potential cause of disease. Moreover, since *pneuma* is present in everything, it is implicit in all the humours. This is confirmed if we consider that a prominent feature of the humours is their ability to flow, to *move*. The author also points out here that wind can be in winter thick and cold, and in summer gentle and calm; so its qualities change with the seasons, or in other words as it mingles with other aspects of nature. This ability is applied to the bodily air; it can mingle with bile or phlegm and cause problems. This is what is discussed in *Breaths* and in *The Sacred Disease*.

The human breath when normal is slightly warm and moist and it moves in a regular cycle or rhythm—qualities that are synonymous with life. Air in the body, when healthy would be the same: slightly warm and moist and moving rhythmically in a cycle. But when imbalanced these qualities in it lessen and it becomes cold, and/or drying, and its movement irregular in some way; or all three of these can be present. It then becomes responsible for destruction of the body, just as the outer air can be violently destructive. This description fits the symptoms seen in melancholy: those of coldness, dryness and various forms of spasms, and tremors and paralyses—derangements of the movement (*Breaths* VIII). Imbalance can also be seen in an excess of

---

188. Jones (1981) vol. II 229, 231 *logismos* is usually translated as reason, and this is usually understood to be the reasoning, intellectualising, analysing and problem-solving faculty in human beings. However, it is also quite possible that the term carried another meaning for the ancients, that of a faculty capable of direct perception of non-physical or what may be called subtle energy or purely spiritual reality. This faculty may be what is recognised by the philosophy of the *Upaniṣads* (cf *Kaṭha Upaniṣad* ii, 9) and the teachings of Christian mystics and of Buddhism and Taoism. Entralgo's discussion of the therapeutic logos in Plato as *epode* leading through *katharsis* and *emmetria* to a *sophrosyne* of the soul, pp. 108-138, suggests the Greeks also recognised this capability in man. Empedocles' *philotes* which made possible a harmonious mingling of the elements may have been a similar vehicle.

air and heat, as in a fever; in the condensation of the moisture in the air of the body as water which then flows out of the body as sweat; or to any part of the body it reaches in excess air becomes the seat of a disease (*Breaths* XIV). Thus wherever it accumulates in excess, it can provoke the other humours, or tissues: phlegm, blood or bile causing phlegmatic symptoms, apoplexy or the sacred disease, epilepsy. In epilepsy it is through its influence on the blood, the embodiment of intelligence, that pneuma causes disturbance, chilling the blood and corrupting it (*Breaths* XIV). This produces a loss of consciousness and a falling. Blood also contains air, so in fevers the extra heat in the blood first vapourises the air in it, then this moisture condenses.

Thus air, in *Breaths*, in effect acts like a humour, a fluid in the body. It is present in the body, it flows. While being necessary to life, normal and healthy, like the traditional humours, it causes its problems when it is excessive, blocked or too cold. It affects vital heat and moisture, consciousness and movement, the very aspects of the organism that we have seen are affected most by excess of the humour, black bile. It has different qualities depending on the season: warm and calm in summer, yet thick and cold in winter, depending on which other element (fire or water), or humour, (phlegm, bile, or blood) it associates with.

Through air mixing with blood, now that the seat of consciousness was, after Empedocles, considered to be located in the heart–lungs, if the blood becomes less and the man is chilled by the coldest humour—melancholy—not only is consciousness altered but the patient, in extreme cases, is also close to death. Such symptoms as those seen in conditions of black bile represent in fact the opposite to man's normal healthy state, both physical and mental—the state associated with life itself: warmth, moisture, consciousness and movement. The opposite of any one or, in worst cases all of these, is associated with particular diseases and even approaching death. Death is marked by the loss of the vital elements and is both what we fear most and associate with deep sadness.

*Diseases IV* and other treatises also associate congestion or blockage of normal water balance in the spleen with melancholy and its qualities of dryness, emaciation and weakness.[189]

In Chapter VII of *Regiment in Acute Diseases* we find air associated with these very imbalances and with movement and mental state. Stoppage of air through the vessels produces pains and fluxes of dark bile: "the vessels being irritated and too dry stretch tight, swell up and attract the fluxes." From this since the blood becomes disordered and the air is no longer able to follow its normal paths through the blood, chills occur as a result of stasis, along with the darkening of the vision, loss of speech, heaviness of the head and convulsions. "From this patients become epileptic or are paralysed... and are dried up because air cannot pass through."[190]

Taking the evidence of these treatises together, it appears that each of the other three humours can affect consciousness by their action on the blood. Bile, as we have seen, arouses irritability and anger; excess phlegm sometimes chills blood, causing loss of consciousness, and sometimes heats it causing inflammations; melancholy brings irregular mental states, something like our nervous breakdown, as well as madness or depression. These connections to blood are part of the concept that air or breath is the vehicle of thought, consciousness and hence life in the body and that (in the body) air is mixed with the blood.

Consideration of the properties of universal and bodily air as described above and a comparison of its effects with those witnessed in diseases associated with the blood and melancholy humour suggest that the model of *Nature of Man* may represent an attempt to account for or incorporate (literally, materialise) cosmic air in the basic make up of human *phusis*. This may be why, in addition to the fact that they were looking for some other "mechanical agent", as Thivel calls it, to explain certain new discoveries about bodily and psychic processes or to refine their older concepts, the physicians appropriated melancholy

189. Lonie (1981) 291-292.
190. Potter (1988) vol. VI 269.

from the popular culture: its characteristics matched the effects of disturbed *pneuma*. Thus although *Nature of Man* does not speak of *pneuma*, its model of the four humours may be a means of incorporating into the medical reasoning the functions of the vital air, perceiving in the blood humour the qualities of air when in its optimal state and in the melancholy humour the qualities of air when it is in a deranged state. In doing so the model simultaneously makes explicit the physician's cognisance of the spirit–mind–body reality of man's essential *phusis*. If so, this would represent in Greek terms the equivalent of Ayurvedic medicine's incorporation of the *prāṇa-vāyu* or vital, cosmic breath or air as the physical *doṣa vāta*. Such a model's inclusion of blood and melancholy would allow the physicians a finer understanding of the processes of change in the body that they were witnessing, and a means of extending this understanding to include the other aspects of the psychic-spiritual spheres of man's *phusis* not previously covered in the earlier bi-polar model.

Thivel seems to regret the emergence of this new model, considering it more fixed and less dynamic than the earlier bi-polar one of phlegm and bile. Others too seem to feel that, as modelled on Empedocles, this is an intrusion of philosophy into medicine which is not healthy, which blocks further progress and development.[191] But this model of the body is even more dynamic, and certainly more comprehensive, or, as we might say today, holistic, since it takes into account not just polarities of heat–cold, moist–dry, phlegm–bile but also even finer nuances of seasons, climates and ages, and more of man's mental, psychological and even spiritual state of health. To do this it incorporates as a humour the most important agent of change, of transformation, and an even more fundamental and universal principle: the life–breath–soul.

Perhaps it is also trying to apply not only Empedocles' root elements but seeking for a bodily presence of Empedocles' agent of their harmonious mingling: love/philotes. Empedocles may

191. Longrigg (1993) 82. Thivel (1981) 77 also finds the latter model of *Nature of Man* too rigid, creating an obstacle to the understanding of being.

have "materialised" air, in the sense that he showed how this universal principle was manifested at the physical level as a substance; this need not mean it lost its non-material or divine qualities. He was also interested in the other aspects of human *phusis*, as well as in the purely physical ones. If the physicians were so profoundly influenced by Empedocles, would not they also have been influenced by other aspects of his thought? Perhaps the bodily *pneuma* becomes for the physicians the embodiment of Empedocles' universal harmonising principle as is suggested by the testimony of the physician Eryximachus at Plato's *Symposium*:

> ...the business of what we call medicine, which is, in a word, the knowledge of the principles of love at work in the body in regard to repletion and evacuation. The most skilful doctor is the doctor who can distinguish between noble and base loves in this sphere, and the man who can cause a body to change the latter for the former, and can implant love in a body which lacks but needs it, and remove it where it already exists, will be a good practitioner. He must be able to bring elements in the body which are most hostile to one another into mutual affections and love; such hostile elements are the opposites hot and cold, wet and dry and the like; it was by knowing how to create love and harmony between these that our forefather Asclepius, as our poets say and as I believe, founded our craft.[192]

## CONCLUSION

If we compare the features of the Greek and Ayurvedic concepts of humours, health–disease and treatment as seen in *Caraka* and *Hippocratic Corpus*, we find much common ground in their understanding of "what man is."

First. Both *doṣas* and humours are bodily manifestations of natural and cosmic elements in the human body. Both *doṣas* and humours are the constituents of the body, along with organs, and other tissues and structures. Both are seen as part of health

192. *The Symposium*, Hamilton (1972) 54-55.

and of disease, that is, they are at the same time constituent elements of the human body when in harmonious balance and the pathogenic factors when this balance is disturbed in some way. In Āyurveda this pathological predisposition is made explicit in that the term *doṣa* itself means defect or fault.

In the Greek conception, from several cosmic elements, including for some thinkers a void (*Diseases IV*, 35), an originally bi-polar explanation of the body constituents and functions was conceived. This became in time a four-fold model, though a concept of a void was retained as an important factor in some treatises. *Nature of Man* speaks of four humours with four corresponding qualities. However, variations on the theme of humours continued to exist. *Ancient Medicine* mentions 'many others' as it mentions tastes, humours and qualities (XV, XVII) and condemns those who only dwell on hot and cold; *Diseases IV* mentions bile as being light, an additional quality to hot and dry. Such evidence suggests that there were at least some strands in the Greek tradition that enumerated more than four qualities. It may be that even more qualities were assumed to be known, though they are not mentioned, as many such qualities can all be derived from the basic four.

*Caraka*, by contrast, enumerates a catalogue of exactly twenty pairs of opposite qualities of the cosmic elements and these are manifested in the bodily *doṣas*. Some *doṣas* share some of these qualities, so that the understanding of how a *doṣa* is imbalanced (and what needs to be done to rebalance it) is much more finely tuned—or some might say complicated—in the case of Āyurveda. In both systems, the humour or *doṣa* is also associated with a particular body organ, function or tissue, though at the same time they are considered to be everywhere in the body. The reservoirs of *Diseases IV* suggest similar concepts among some Greek physicians.

Phlegm as representing the vital fluid of the body, when normal constitutes health, but when it is contracted/dried out or otherwise deranged it causes epilepsy or, in some treatises, other forms of mental illness as it becomes transformed into melancholy. This seems an interesting point of similarity to the contrast in Āyurveda between vāta and the vital essence *ojas.* The symptoms of aggravated *vāta,* low *ojas* include—the mental imbalance and loss of movement and/or weakness, the emaciation are almost exactly the symptoms associated with the melancholy humour. The qualities of *vāta* and low *ojas* are the opposites to those of phlegm and abundant cerebral-spinal marrow. It appears that each system recognises the same basic vital elements with corresponding qualities but each configures them and the dynamics between these in a slightly different way, commensurate perhaps with their different geographical and climatic conditions.

Second. Both systems see a humour or *doṣa* as capable of moving in the body, flowing out of their main sites, mixing with other humours or *doṣas* or with tissues or *dhātus,* dissolving and spreading to other parts of the body where it concentrates, or undergoes further change and causes further imbalance and possibly transforming into another condition. Again this process is much made more explicit and detailed in *Caraka.*

Third. Both models recognise a divine aspect to creation and see the mental-spiritual aspects of humans as also part of the qualities of the humours or *doṣas.* The patient's state of mind is an important factor in the disease and its treatment. In *Caraka,* the divine and psychic takes a very prominent role and there is a great deal of text devoted to it. In the Hippocratic *Corpus* it is much less apparent, though it is definitely present.

Fourth. Both models recognise that humans can be grouped according to shared physical and mental features into constitutional types based on their balance of humours or *doṣas.* The *phusis* or *prakṛti* is understood thoroughly within the context or matrix of the wider world: the seasons, climate, habitation, food sources, waters and age. This again is worked out in much more detail in *Caraka.* The role of the physician is conceived similarly in each system: to recognise the constitutional type, which of the specific *doṣas* or humours that are out of balance in that person and the specific tissues, organs or functions of the body these humours are affecting and treat accordingly. Treatments are along very similar lines, though there is much more text as regards both drugs and treatments in *Caraka* so we have a clearer idea of what was done.

Fifth. Both models employ concepts of like to like and antagonism of opposites in their explanations of disease. Both employ similar therapeutic methods, emphasising diet, lifestyle and exercise regimens, but also employing drugs (herbs, animal substances and minerals). The methods themselves are also similar, both systems valuing 'cleansing' therapies: purgation, emesis to restore balance to the digestive tract, fomentation and vapour baths to promote release through sweat, oleation and massage, blood letting to release excess of blood. The aim is to mature or return the humour or *doṣa* to its normal state, return it to its normal site in the body and cleanse the excess of the humour from the body through eliminative channels.

In both traditions there is a dominant, perhaps an older model of humours – bi-polar in the case of the *Corpus*, tri-polar in the case of *Caraka*, but there is also some flexibility within this. In *Caraka* we find blood acting in effect like a humour, while in the *Corpus* some treatises conceive of three and some of four humours. These variations could represent different strands of tradition or the varying approaches of different physicians based on their particular experience and reasonings. In *Caraka* these are ultimately harmonised or homogenised, while in the *Corpus*, the differences remain outstanding—at least until Galen imposes his order on them centuries later.

Sixth. Both models give fundamental importance to the concept of cosmic air underlying all other natural processes, as embodying the life-soul-consciousness in the body. Each incorporates this into one of their fundamental constituents: *Vāta doṣa* and *prāṇa* in the case of Āyurveda. In the *Corpus* this is done differently by different authors. Melancholy may be the vehicle for the author of *Nature of Man* to express the characteristics of deranged biological air. The author of *Breaths* is explicit in describing the functions and effects of bodily air as *pneuma or phusa*.

Seven. Considering the evidence of *Diseases IV*, both models also include the idea of void, or space (*aither, ākāśa*) in their understanding of the natural world. However, in the *Corpus* this only appears in this one treatise in regard to gestation of the embryo. Still, since gestation of the human embryo may have been modeled on, or be a reflection in the individual of the cosmic process of creation, this may hold more significance than at first appears. It may have been part of the knowledge of authors of other treatises, though it is not mentioned by them as the subject at hand in the treatise does not call for it. In the Sāṃkhya philosophy as reflected in *Caraka* this component of creation is included and given a definite sphere of activity, sound, though, as with the *Corpus*, it is not otherwise given importance.

In other ways there are significant contrasts between *Caraka* and *Corpus*. In *Caraka* a significant proportion of the chapters are devoted to an explanation of the origins and nature not only of man and but also, quite explicitly, the soul. Yet we also find that by comparison, the proportion of text dealing with a detailed explanation of the relationship of the *doṣa* and *dhātus* to these cosmic forces is relatively small. Again here too, the knowledge about the relationship between the cosmic elements and the bodily *doṣas* is not explicitly set out but is more implicit, or seems to have been more or less taken for granted.[193] In the *Corpus*, while there is definitely recognition of the divine throught the concept of nature, of soul and some recognition of the mental–emotional aspects involved it is meagre compared to the detailed discussions we find in *Caraka*. Comparatively little attention is paid to this aspect relative to other subjects in the treatises. This may be because works including such topics were lost, or were of particular interest only to certain types of physicians (such as those responsible for the *Oath*, for example). On the other hand, in the *Corpus* we have much more evidence of the detailed observations being carried out (e.g. the *Epidemics*), records of clinical notes so that we have a record of the thoughts of individual physicians and can hear their individual voices. In *Caraka* physicians are exhorted to be acutely observant but we have no similar evidence of their clinical notes. They hold

193. Chattopadhyaya (1979) e.g. 263-265. He explains the 'religious' parts of *Caraka* as being interpolations into a medical corpus to satisfy the demands of the powerful Brahmin influence.

symposia and propound differing views on subjects, but ultimately these are harmonised. Still, the fact that they are aired indicates differences among the physicians or different strands of traditions.

We have seen that in the fifth and fourth centuries, in the Greek world, there were several and varying explanations of the nature of man put forward by the natural philosophers and by the medical thinkers, though each explanation aims to explain the same phenomena: life, heat, moisture, cold, dryness and movement and their manifestations as health or disease. These gradually became systematised into a four-humoural, four-quality model of man and his world. We have seen that in *Caraka*, although primarily one system, Sāṃkhya forms the basis for the organisation of information there are also variant elements which suggest there were in fact a diversity of ideas in the tradition, representing perhaps even "layers" of traditions. In a sense in the *Corpus* we can witness a process of development and change, through argumentation and competition among different traditions, and this may shed some light on possible ways the same process happened in Ayurvedic tradition culminating in *Caraka*. While each tradition exhibits variations and exceptions to the 'rule'—for example, blood in the case of Āyurveda, water in the case of the Hippocratic *Corpus*—both systems eventually moved towards one dominant model: a tripartite one in the case of Āyurveda, a four-fold one in the case of Greek medicine.

CHAPTER 5

# DISCUSSION

This book has examined the origins of European medicine as recorded in the Hippocratic *Corpus* in the light of what is now termed 'holistic medicine.' It has been recognised that the medical works were closely related to, although in some ways also different from, Greek philosophical thought of the fifth and sixth centuries B.C. While from a scientific point of view this close connection has been seen as in some ways negative, from the point of view of a holistic practitioner, it is very positive. The reverence for nature and the perception of it as a vital force operating within the human body and its environment is what provides a holistic context to the art of medicine. We have found that some key ideas of holistic medicine, about harmony and balance among different components and forces, about health and disease, about the healing process and about the roles of patient and physician in that process, spring from this philosophical grounding. Viewing the *Corpus* from the standpoint of Āyurveda has helped us to appreciate how the theory and practice of ancient physicians was grounded in just such a philosophical context. We have seen how this context informed the way the physicians approached the treatment of disease and restoration of health through the model of the humours and as applied in the use of regimen (diet, exercise, lifestyle) and medicines. Their practices were the result of reasoning applied to experience. While many of them are not applicable today, on the evidence of similar practices still extant in Āyurveda, many others are capable of application in a contemporary holistic setting, and are being used. The valuable asset of a philosophical grounding, capable of relating all the different factors of the patient's experience, is probably one of the factors that draws the public to holistic medicine today.

This is not to imply that using a holistic approach is to be non-scientific. Neither the public nor practitioners desire this. The ancient Greeks and Indians laid the foundations of scientific enquiry and valued most highly the application of reason to an understanding of existence. But holistic does mean to maintain the perspective of the whole while examining the parts, not to limit the understanding to only the measurable, material level, but to take account even of the operation of non-material elements within the physical realm.

The field of complementary and alternative medicine today and especially the numerous disciplines within it can appear to be lacking any common principles and philosophy. Indeed this was the view of the British Medical Association's report "Complementary Medicine: New Approaches to Good Practice".[1] Among the different practitioners too there may be a lack of awareness of common threads among them. An understanding of the Hippocratic *Corpus* helps us to realise there is a common foundation for disciplines as seemingly diverse as herbal medicine, massage, naturopathy, aromatherapy, osteopathy and chiropractic, nutritional and dietary therapy, relaxation, visualisation and stress management techniques, perhaps even humanistic counselling and flower essences. Even the relatively new therapy of cranial –sacral work has a resonance with the ancient practices which recognised the importance of the cerebral spinal fluid and its intimate involvement with other body functions and processes. Here again the comparison with Āyurveda can be helpful. We find that its founding principles underpin its several specialised therapeutic interventions: dietary therapy, herbal medicine and pharmacy, massage, gemstone and colour therapy, mantra and visualisation techniques. All these co-exist under its umbrella. If we, as Western holistic practitioners, could appreciate that each of us is also practising one of many strands within a tradition based on common insights, common principles and philosophy dating back more than two thousand years, it would lend strength to our current efforts at self-regulation, the setting of standards

1. *Integrated Health Care* (1997) 3.

and at establishing our professions within an "integrated" national health care system.

Highlighting the salient holistic features of Hippocratic medicine from the myriad of details and varieties of subject matter and authors in the *Corpus* makes it clear that there is a substantial body of knowledge and experience available from this source of Western medicine. The results of the analyses here suggest several points for exploration into possible applications in contemporary practice, or for further research.

Many practitioners, for example herbalists, are seeking to re-weave the fragmented strands of our history into a useful body of theory and practice applicable today alongside contributions from science. Such an effort has formed part of the work of Simon Mill's *Out of the Earth* and Peter Holmes' *Energetics of Western Herbs*. Most recently,. Graeme Tobyn's *Culpeper's Medicine, A Practice of Western Holistic Medicine* has re-evaluated Culpeper as an important figure in this tradition and records his dependence on Hippocratic concepts. This book is a very welcome step in the reappraisal by practitioners of our own traditions, though a more thorough grounding in the actual Hippocratic *Corpus* and its context is important. For it is difficult to understand fully the work of Galen, Paracelsus and Culpeper without understanding this crucial source of so much of their own work, from which they evolved or reacted to.[2] In addition, for naturopaths and dietary therapists, it is again advantageous to know about the wealth of material and guiding principles on diet and regimen in the *Corpus*. Like our ancient predecessors, practitioners today essentially seek to re-establish the body's internal harmony, though cur repertoire of therapies benefits from progress and development over the centuries.

If we ask if there is anything in the *Corpus* which is relevant to a modern holistic practice we find that several of the key concepts of Greek medicine are present in a contemporary form. Its understanding of the mind–body nexus as constitutional types and their predispositions corresponds, for example, to that of

2. Other components of the sources, of course, are also very important, e.g. women's healing traditions and temple or religious medicine.

Meyers–Briggs personality types (e.g. the A-type being predisposed to heart disease).[3] Hippocratic–Galenic constitutional types, being more holistic, can be even more useful as indicators of potential health problems and as guides to the most advantageous treatments and lifestyle habits for the individual in his or her particular environment. In another sphere, the guidelines in the *Corpus* on fasting and mono-diets to re-establish the balance in the digestive intestinal functions, on re-examination, may have lessons in the treatment of food allergies, malabsorption and excess conditions that predispose to infections, weakness or candidiasis. In fact, it seems it is essentially these guidelines that form the basis of some dietary therapies today. In herbal medicine it may be worth a new look at some of the herbal remedies recorded in the *Corpus* (and subsequently those in Galen and later physicians) which, while not present in current treatment protocols, might suggest 'new' uses of our Western *materia medica* in the modern practice.

Current bio-medical research on the effects of mental states on immunity, and on the processes of humoural immunity, i.e. the fluid-mediated immune responses, also finds resonances in the concepts of the ancient physicians. Immunology is becoming one of the most important components of bio-medicine at the beginning of the twenty-first century. In the light of this, the inferences coupled with experience which led the Hippocratic physicians to recognise the primary importance of the state of the body's fluids to its health and vitality and to recovering from disease are proved to be extremely sophisticated and perceptive. From the vantage point of the beginning of the twenty-first century replete with extensive and detailed knowledge of the body and the ability to manipulate it with chemical technology, the humoural model can look extremely naive, merely "theoretical",

3. Sigerist, citing the work of psychiatrist E. Kretschmer in the 1920s, foreshadowed this when he commented "modern psychosomatic studies...have shown that most of these ancient constitutional types are not fictitious, not the result of a desire to systematise vague observations, but are very real and may be described in scientific terms." (1961) 325.

based on unproved assumptions and relatively ineffective. The ancient understanding of physiology and pathology came from a time when knowledge of anatomy was rudimentary and it lacks the detail and precision of current knowledge. Yet this did not prevent the physicians from realising that numerous bodily processes are mediated through its fluids, especially its immunity and strength of self-preservation, and that these are interconnected with its mental–emotional states. They found that these humours and psychological states could be influenced by the physician and the patient himself and were certain they are worth parity of attention in treatment.[4] Perhaps their situation forced physicians to appreciate and make use of other ways of understanding the body, ways that have not lost their relevance to holistic practice today.

It has been extremely interesting to compare these two traditional medicine systems. While acknowledging the differences between them, the lasting impression is that there is a great amount which they hold in common. Further study is warranted. For example, a study documenting how the basic Hippocratic ideas were developed, refined, altered (or abandoned) by Galen and subsequent practitioners would be valuable. Some Classics scholars have drawn on anthropological studies of pre-literate cultures to aid our understanding of the Greek mind.[5] The findings of this book would suggest that our understanding might also be served by a comparative study of representative social groups within Indian culture (Hindu or Muslim). It also would be illuminating to understand why the Greek system seemed to be unable to accommodate new scientific thought and fell into disrepute. Again here, Ayurvedic medicine's evolution through contact with colonial Western medicine may make a useful comparison. Another interesting

---

4. This important interplay between hormones–fluid secretions carried by another fluid, blood, mediated to cells via intersticial lymph fluid with an important psychological component—and immunity is increasingly being studied today, as the new discipline of "psycho–neuro–immunology" shows. See Nutton (1993) 282 and his reference to Siegal (1968) and Brooks *et al.* (1962).
5. For example, Dodds (1951) and Sallares (1991).

topic suggested is a comparison of the philosophical systems of ancient India and Greece.

Like the early physicians, those early thinkers were attempting to explain their perception of reality. The Hippocratic and Ayurvedic physicians chose different terms to try to convey their concepts according to their different traditions, geography and climate. Yet the experience which generated the concepts, that of the human body–mind–spirit whole, was the same.

# GLOSSARY

## AYURVEDIC TERMS

*agni* : biological fire, the fire of digestion but also the digestive fire that allows for the creation of each tissue in the body in the process of tissue nutrition.

*Agniveśa* : one of the disciples of the sage Ātreya Punarvasu. According to tradition, the catalyst for *Caraka Saṃhitā* was when Ātreya asked his six disciples to compile his teachings on medicine, the relief of suffering and how to live a long and healthy life. Agniveśa's compilation was chosen as the best. The *Caraka Saṃhitā* is a redaction of Agniveśa's teaching, with later additions and alterations.

*ahaṃkāra* : ego or sense of individual self.

*asthi* : see *dhātu*.

*ātman* : another name for the individual soul within the body.

*Brahman* : universal soul, god.

*buddhi* : intellect.

*cetanā* : thought or consciousness.

*dhātu* : tissue or tissue element. The body has seven tissues: *rasa* or chyle juice (the first product of food digestion,); *rakta* or blood, blood elements; *māṃsa* or muscle; *medas* or fat; *asthi* or bone; *majjan* or marrow; *śukra* or semen/reproductive fluids.

*doṣa* : literally a fault. In medicine it refers to the three biological forces which are the components of the human body. Each of the three *doṣas* is made of two of the five great elements, space, air, fire, water and earth.

*guṇas* : sometimes called the mental *doṣas,* the three *guṇas* represent tendencies or attributes of the mind. *Sattva* indicates clarity, understanding, calmness, compassion, love. *Rajas* indicates activity, desire, will to action, assertion. *Tamas* indicates inertia, heaviness, dullness, lack of understanding.

*kapha* : the biological *doṣa* deriving from the elements water and earth. It embodies the principle of coolness and moisture in the body and is responsible for the production of fluids, lubrication, formation of flesh, strength and stability. It is reflected in the emotions of envy, attachment and greed but also of compassion, forgiveness and love.

*karma* : literally action. *The law of karma* refers to the concept that souls reincarnate to enjoy the fruits of their actions in a previous life.

*Mahābhūtas* : the five great (*mahā*) elements (*bhūta*) out of which the physical creation is formed. These are space *(ākāśa),* air (*vāyu*), fire (*tejas*), water (*jala*) and earth *(pṛthvi*).

*majjan* : see *dhātu*.

*māṃsa* : see *dhātu*.

*manas* : mind.

*medas* : see *dhātu*.

*mokṣa* : liberation. From the ascetic point of view, the object of life is for the soul to gain liberation from its attachment to the mind and body in order to return to its unity with the cosmic or universal soul, *Brahma*.

*nāḍī* : a channel, a *srota*.

*pitta* : the biological *doṣa* deriving from fire and water (liquidity). It embodies the principle of heat in the body and is responsible for metabolism and catabolic processes, the formation of blood, tissue combustion, and intelligence. It is reflected in the emotions of anger, jealousy and hate but also of self-protection and defence.

*prajñāparādha* : offence against wisdom.

*prakṛti* : primal nature out of which the physical universe is created; also the individual nature of each person in terms of the balance of the three *doṣas,* one's basic constitutional type.

*prāṇa* : vital air. *Caraka* gives five in the body: incoming, upward moving, balanced, downward moving, sideways or outward moving.

*puruṣa* : according to *Caraka* it is the "empirical soul", or that soul from Brahma which is embodied in the creation to experience it. It is also called the mind–soul–body combination, or sentient being, for which the veda of long life is written. The soul itself is said to be devoid of pathogenicity, to be the cause of consciousness and to be eternal.

*rajas* : see *guṇas*.

*rakta* : see *dhātu*.

*rasa* : see *dhātu*.

*Sāṃkhya* : a school of philosophy whose sources probably date from the three centuries before Christ but whose extant texts date from 100 B.C. to A.D. 200. Their content reflects a great development in analytical enquiry into the evolution of creation and the nature and place of mankind within it. The discourse on these subjects in *Caraka* are closely related to Sāṃkhya and other schools of this period. Sāṃkhya means account, enumeration, or discrimination.

*sattva* : see *guṇas*.

*srotas* : channels of circulation. These are not quite the same as blood vessels, but are conceived as channels through which dosas circulate throughout the body and to the organs.

*śukra* : see *dhātu*.

*tamas* : see *guṇas*.

*tanmātra* : the five subtle elements, the precursors of the five gross or physical elements, existing in a subtle energetic form.

*Upaniṣads* : literally 'sitting near devotedly', or 'secret teaching'. There are one hundred and light texts preserved, ten principal ones, but their individual authors, the *ṛṣis* or sages, are unknown. The authors have recorded their insights, through visions and spiritual experience, about the nature of god and the way to liberate the soul to find union with god.

*vāta* : the biological *doṣa* deriving from the elements of space and air. It embodies the principles of air and movement and is responsible for all sensation, movements, rhythms in the body. It is reflected in the emotions of fear and anxiety, but also in sensitivity and awareness.

*vāyu* : wind, air; also the name of the god of wind Vāyu. Embodied as *prāṇa,* the vital air or *vāta,* the air *doṣa*.

*veda* : knowledge. "āyur veda" means knowldge or science of longevity or how to maintain health and live long, which includes treatment of disease.

*Vedas* : four ancient literary works (1500–1400 B.C.). They are collections of hymns to the deities, mostly gods of nature of the Indo-European tribes who migrated to north-west India. The fourth veda, the Atharva, differs from the other three. It contains charms and spells used by ordinary people, for example to ward off or cure diseases. Atharva thus records much information on the magico–religious practices for healing which predate Āyurveda, and which to some extent still exist in India. Although the root 'veda' is part of the word 'āyurveda', Āyurveda as a rational system of medicine is quite different from the Vedas and should not be confused with them.

*Vaiśeṣika* : another of the six orthodox systems of philosophy in Classical India (the latter half of the first millennium B.C.). It is different from Sāṃkhya and other schools, especially in its doctrine of "viśeṣa", or eternally distinct nature of nine fundamental substances (ether, air, fire, water, earth, mind, time, space and soul). Some of its concepts are also found in *Caraka.*

*yukti* : reasoning or rational application. A term employed in *Caraka* referring, for example, to how the physician can know the effect of a drug. He must reason or take into account that this is determined by all the various interrelated factors involved in the situation—the condition of the patient, his age, the season, time of day, emotional state, etc. It seems similar to the concept of medical reasoning *iatrikos logismos* among the Greek medical writers.

## GREEK TERMS

| | | |
|---|---|---|
| *apostasis* | : | an abcess, collection of morbid matter/ humour in a particular place in the body until it can be excreted. |
| *clyster* | : | enema. |
| *dunamis* | : | power, faculty, energy. |
| *oxymel* | : | a medicinal mixture of vinegar and honey. |
| *hydromel* | : | a medicinal blend of water and honey. |
| *ptisane* | : | barley gruel. It was prepared in several ways, for example, thin (strained) or thick. |
| *perissomata* | : | food residues from poor digestion that imbalance the body. |
| *krasis (kresis in Ionian Greek)* | : | mixing, blending compounding. |
| *krisis* | : | the turning point in the course of a disease, usually fever, when the patient begins to recover. It could be good or not quite complete, therefore not fully turning the condition towards healing. |
| *pepsis* | : | coction or cooking, the chief means by which humours or other factors are blended and harmonised. |

# APPENDIX

## Origin of Man According to *Carakasaṃhitā*

| Brahman/*Puruṣa* | *Prakṛti* |
|---|---|
| (Self, eternal and not subject to change)[1] | (undifferentiated primal matter, eternal and subject to change) with three constituents, the guṇas: light-illuminating, moving, and dense-heavy. |

| *Buddhi* (individual)/*Mahat* (cosmic)[2] | *Ahaṃkāra*[2] |
|---|---|
| (intellect, capacity for wisdom, decider between truth and non-truth) | (ego, self reference, individuator, I-maker) |

| **Five Faculties action** | **Faculty of thought, *Manas*** | **Five Faculties of sense** | **Six *Dhātus*, i.e. the Five Gross of Elements**[2] |
|---|---|---|---|
| (motor organs) | (ordinary mental activities) | | (*mahābhūtas+cetanā*) |
| speaking | mind | hearing | *ākāśa*, ether |
| grasping | | touching | *vāyu*, air |
| walking | | seeing | *tejas*, fire |
| evacuation | | tasting | *jala*, water |
| procreation | | smelling | *pṛthvī*, earth |
| | | | *cetanā, consciousness* |

Total: twenty-four elements

From the great elements are formed the *doṣas* and *dhātus:*
**Three *doṣas*:** *vāta, pitta, kapha*.
**Seven *dhātus*:** *rasa, rakta, māṃsa, medas, asthi, majjan, śukra*.
Their quintessence is ***ojas***, vitality.[3]

---

1. "There is also *Puruṣa*, for had it not been so there would been not birth, death, bondage or salvation." "*Puruṣa* comprises six *dhātus* (elements), viz. five *mahābhūtas* and consciousness (*cetanā*). Even the element of consciousness alone constitutes *Puruṣa*" (Śārīrasthāna I, 16). "According to another classification, *Puruṣa* comprises twenty-four *dhātus*, i.e. mind (*manas*), ten *indriyas* (five sensory and five motor organs), five objects of sense-organs and *Prakṛti* [consisting of eight *dhātus*, viz. five *mahābhūtas*, *ahaṃkāra*, *mahat* and *avyakta* (primordial element) (*prakṛti*/nature) ]" (Śārīrasthāna I, 17). "The combination of the above mentioned twenty-four elements [or categories] is known as *Puruṣa*." (Śārīrasthāna I, 35). "The contact of *Puruṣa* with twenty-four elements continues so long as He is influenced by *rajas* and *tamas*. The moment He gets rid of *rajas* and *tamas*, he is freed from contacts by virtue of the dominance of sattva" (Śārīrasthāna I, 36). "The Absolute Soul [Brahman] is beginningless and as such is eternal. The Empirical Soul (i.e. the combination of 24 elements) being caused by something is not so, i.e. it has a beginning and is ephemeral" (Śārīrasthāna I, 59).
2. "The intellect (*buddhi*) originates from avyakta (*prakṛti* /primordial nature), ego (*ahaṃkāra*) from intellect (*buddhi*) and five *mahābhūtas* (viz. *ākāśa*, etc.) from ego. The Empirical Soul *(Puruṣa)* thus manifested in its entirety is regarded as born" (Śārīrasthāna, I, 66-67). "Mind is the connecting link which connects the Soul with the physical body" (Śārīrasthāna III, 13).
3. I am indebted to Anne Glazier for help in compiling this scheme. For further information, see *A History of Indian Philosophy*, Surendranath Dasgupta, Vol. I, 213 ff.

# BIBLIOGRAPHY

## I. ANCIENT WORKS


*Caraka Saṃhitā* Sharma, R.K., and Dash, B.V. (trans.) Varanasi Chowkhamba 1985.

*Enquiry into Plants* Theophrastus vol. I and II Holt, A. (trans.) London William Heinemann 1916, 1968.

*The Greek Herbal of Dioscorides: Edited by a Byzantine A.D.* 512 *Englished by John Goodyer A.D.* 1655 Gunther, R.T (ed.) Newyork Hafner Publishing 1968.

*Geographia* Strabo Jones, H.L.(trans.) Loeb Classical Library London Heinemann 1949.

*Hippocrate* tomes II and V Jouanna, J. (trans.) Paris Societe D'Edition "Les Belles Lettres" 1990.

*Hippocrate Oevre complet* Vol. 8 Littré, E. Amsterdam Adolf M. Hakkert 1962.

*Hippocrates* Loeb Classical Library Cambridge MA Harvard University Press London William Heinemann Ltd.

Jones, W.H.S. (trans.) Volume I. *Ancient Medicine; Airs, Waters, Places; Epidemics* I; *Epidemics* III; *The Oath; Precepts; Nutriment* 1972.

Jones, W.H.S. (trans.) Volume II. *Prognostic; Regimen in Acute Diseases; The Sacred Disease; The Art; Breaths; Law; Decorum; Physician* (Chapter 1); *Dentition* 1981.

Withington, E.T. (trans.) Volume III. *On Wounds in the Head; In the Surgery; On Fractures; On Joints; Instruments of Reduction* 1968.

Jones, W.H.S. (trans.) Volume IV. *Nature of Man; Regimen in Health; Humours; Aphorisms; Regimen* I; *Regimen* II; *Regimen* III; *Regimen* IV/ *Dreams; Heracleitus: On the Universe* 1979.

Potter, P. (trans.) Volume V. *Affections; Diseases* I; *Diseases* II 1988.

Potter, P. (trans.) Volume VI. *Diseases* III; *Internal Affections; Regimen in Acute Diseases* 1988.

Smith, W.D. (trans.) Volume VII. *Epidemics* 2; *Epidemics* 4; *Epidemics* 5; *Epidemics* 6 1994.

Potter, P. (trans.) Volume VIII. *Places in Man; Glands; Fleshes; Prorrhetic* 1; *Prorrhetic* 2; *Physician; Use of Liquids; Ulcers; Haemorrhoids and Fistulas* 1995.

*Hippocratic Writings* Lonie I.M Withington, E.T. Chadwick J. and Mann W.N. (trans.) with introduction by G.E.R. Lloyd Harmondsworth, Middex Penguin 1986.

*The Medical Writings of the Anonymous Londinensis* Jones, W.H.S. (trans.) Cambridge Cambridge University Press 1947.

*On the Parts of Medicine, On Cohesive Causes, On Regimen in Acute Diseases in Accordance with the Theories of Hippocrates* (Corpus Medicorum Graecorum) Galen Lyons, M. (trans.) Berlin Akademie-Verlag 1969.

*The Symposium,* Plato Hamilton, W. (trans.) Harmondsworth, Middex Penguin 1951.

*Sacred Books of the East* vol. XXV *The Laws of Manu 1886;* vol. XII *The Śatapatha Brāhmaṇa* section I 1882; vol. XLIV *The Śatapatha Brāhmaṇa* section V 1891 series edited by F. Max Müller Oxford University Press.

*The Thirteen Principal Upanishads* Hume, R.E. (trans.) London Oxford University Press 1921, Delhi 1983.

*The Charmides* Plato Watt, D. (trans.) in Saunders, T.J. (ed.) *Early Socratic Dialogues* Harmondsworth, Middex Penguin 1987.

## II. MODERN WORKS

Bonnard, Andre *Greek Civilisation* New York Macmillan Co. 1962.

Bourgey, L. and Jouanna, J. (eds.) *La Collection hippocratique et so role dans l'histoire de la medecine: colloque de Strasbourg* Leiden Brill 1975.

Brooks, C.M., Gilbert, J.L., Levey, H.A., Curtis, D.R. *Humours, Hormones and Neurosecretions* New York State University of New York 1962.

Burkett, Walter *Greek Religion* Oxford Basil Blackwell 1990

Burkett, Walter *Lore and Science in Ancient Pythagoreanism* Cambridge, MA. Harvard University Press 1972.

Burnet, John *Early Greek Philosophy* London Adam and Charles Black, Ltd. 1892, 1963.

Burnet, John "Philosophy" in Livingston, R.W. (ed.) *The Legacy of Greece* Oxford The Clarendon Press 1922, p. 57-95.

Bynum, W.F. and Porter, R. *Companion Encyclopedia of the History of Medicine* 2 vols. London Routledge 1993.

Clendening, Logan (compiler) *Source Book of Medical History* New York Dover Publications, Inc. 1960.

Chattopadhyaya, Debiprasad *Science and Society in Ancient India* Calcutta Research India Publications 1979.

Conrad, L.I., Neve, M., Nutton, V., Porter, R., Wear, A. *The Western Medical Tradition* : 800B.C.-A.D. 1800 Cambridge Cambridge University Press 1995.

Christopher, John *The School of Natural Healing* Provo, UT Bi-World Publishers 1976.

Cousins, Norman *Anatomy of an illness as perceived by the patient: Reflections on healing and regeneration* New York Bantam Books 1981.

Coward, Rosalind *The Whole Truth: The Myth of Alternative Health* London Faber and Faber 1989.

Craik, Elizabeth "Diet, diaita and dietetics" in Powell, Anton (ed.) *The Greek World* London Routledge 1995.

Craik, Elizabeth "Hippokratic Diaita" in Wilkins, John; Harvey, David and Dodson, Mike (eds.) *Food in Antiquity: Studies in Ancient Society and Culture* Exeter Exeter University Press 1995

Dasgupta, Surendranath, *A History of Indian Philosophy* Vol.I Cambridge Cambidge University Press 1957.

Demand, Nancy *Birth, Death and Motherhood in Classical Greece* Baltimore Johns Hopkins University Press 1994.

Demand, Nancy "Monuments Midwives and Gynecology" in van der Eijk P. J., Horstmanshoff, H.J.F., Schrijvers, P.H. (eds.) *Ancient Medicine in its Socio-Cultural Context*, vol.I Amsterdam Rodopi 1995 pp. 275-290.

Detienne, Marcel *The Gardens of Adonis: Spices in Greek Mythology* Lloyd J. (trans' from French) Princeton, NJ Princeton University Press 1994.

Dodds, E.R. *The Greeks and the Irrational* Berkeley, CA University of California Press 1951.

Edelstein, Ludwig *Ancient Medicine: Selected papers of Ludwig Edelstein* Baltimore London Johns Hopkins University Press 1967.

Featherstone, Cornelia and Forsyth, Lori *Medical Marriage: The new partnership between orthodox and complementary medicine* London Findhorn Press 1997.

Filliozat, Jean *The Classical Doctrine of Indian Medicine* Chanana D.R. (Eng. trans. from french) Delhi Munshiram Manoharlal 1964.

Frawley, David *Ayurvedic Healing Course* (Three Parts) American Institute of Vedic Studies Santa Fe New Mexico 1991.

Furley, David J., and Wilkie, J.S. *Galen on Respiration and the Arteries* Princeton, NJ Princeton University Press 1982.

Grant, Doris and Joice, Jean *Food Combining for Health: Don't Mix Foods That Fight* London Thorsons-Harper Collins 1991.

Griggs, Barbara *Green Pharmacy: The story of western herbal medicine* London Jill Norman and Hobhonse 1981.

Guthrie, W.K.C. *A History of Greek Philosophy*, Vols. I-VI Cambridge Cambridge University Press 1962–1981.

Haeckel, E. *Last Words on Evolution: A popular retrospect and summary* McCabe, J. (trans.) from the 2nd edn. London A.Owen 1906.

Hanson, A.E. "Paidopoiia: Metaphors for conception, abortion and gestation in the Hippocratic Corpus" in van der Eijk, P.J., Horstmanshoff, H.J.F., Schrijvers, P. H. *(eds.) Ancient Medicine in its Socio-Cultural Context*, vol. I Amsterdam Rodopi 1995.

Hanson, A.E. "The medical writers's woman" in Halperin, Davis M., Winkler, John J., Zeitlin, Fion I. (eds.) *Before Sexuality: The construction of erotic experience in the ancient Greek world* Princeton, NJ Princeton University Press 1990.

Hanson, A.E. "Conception, Gestation, and the Origin of Female Nature in the *Corpus Hippocraticum*" *Helios* vol. 19, 1992 pp. 31-71.

Holmes, Peter *The Energetics of Western Herbs* Berkeley, CA NatTrop 1993.

Hornblower S., Spawforth A. *The Oxford Classical Dictionary* Oxford Oxford University Press 1996.

Huffman, Carl A. *Philolaus of Croton: Pythagorean and Presocratic: A Commentary on the Fragment and Testimonia with Interpretive Essays* Cambridge Cambridge University Press 1993.

Hussey, Edward "Ionian Enquiries: the Pre-Socratic basis of Science", in Powel, A. (ed.) *The Greek World* London Routledge 1995 pp. 530-549.

*Integrated Health Care: A Discussion Document* The Foundation for Integrated Medicine 1997.

Irwin, Terence *Classical Thought* Oxford Oxford University Press 1989.

Joly, Robert "Le systeme cnidien des humeurs", in Bourgey L., Jouanna J. (eds.) *La Collection hippocratique et son role dans l'historie de la medecine* collouque de Strasbourg Leiden Brill 1975. pp. 107-127.

Jolly, Julius *Indian Medicine* New Delhi Munshiram Manoharlal 1994.

Jones, W.H.S. *Malaria and Greek History* Manchester Manchester University Press 1909.

Kingsley, Peter *Ancient Philosophy, Mystery and Magic* Oxford University Press (Clarendon) 1995.

Kirk, G.S. (ed.) *The Presocratic Philosophers: A critical history with a selection of texts* Cambridge Cambridge University Press 1983.

Kirchfeld, Friedhelm and Boyd, Wade *Nature Doctors: Pioneers in naturopathic medicine* E. Palestine, Ohio Buckeye Naturopathic Press 1994.

Kuhn, Thomas S. *The Structure of Scientific Revolutions* Chicago IL University of Chicago Press 1962, 1970.

Lain Entralgo, Pedro *The Therapy of the Word in Classical Antiquity* New Haven CT Yale University Press 1970.

Larson, James Gerald and Bhattacharya, Ram Shankar *Encyclopedia of Indian Philosophies, Vol. IV: Sāṃkyha, A Dualist Tradition in Indian Philosophy* Princeton, NJ Princeton University Press 1987.

Lele, R.D. *Ayurveda and Modern Medicine* Bombay Bharatiya Vidya Bhavan 1986.

Liddell, H.G. and Scott, R. *A Greek-English Lexicon* Ninth Edition Oxford Oxford University Press 1968.

Livingstone, R.W. (ed.) *The Legacy of Greece* Oxford The Clarendon Press 1922.

Lloyd, G.E.R. "Introduction" in Lloyd, G.E.R. (ed.) *Hippocratic Writings* Chadwick J., Mann W.N. (trans. from the Greek) London and New York Penguin 1978.

Lloyd, G.E.R. *Magic, Reason and Experience: Studies on the origin and development of Greek Science* Cambridge and New York Cambridge University Press 1979.

Lloyd, G.E.R. *Early Greek Science: Thales to Aristotle* London Chatto and Windus 1982.

Lloyd, G.E.R. *Revolutions of Wisdom: Studies on the claims and practice of ancient Greek Science* Berkeley, CA University of California Press 1987.

Lloyd, G.E.R. *Methods and Problems in Greek Science* Cambridge and New York Cambridge University Press 1991.

Lloyd, G.E.R. "Adversaries and Authorities" *Proceedings of the Cambridge Philological Society* No. 40 1994 pp. 27-48.

Longrigg, James *Greek Rational Medicine* London Routledge 1993.

Lonie, Iain M. *The Hippocratic Treatises "On Generation", "The Nature of the Child, Diseases IV"* Ars Medica II 7 New York Walter de Gruyter 1981.

Luce, J.V. *An Introduction to Greek Philosophy* London Thames and Hudson 1992.

Lust, John *The Herb Book* New York Bantam Books 1974.

Majno, Guido *The Healing Hand: Man and wound in the ancient world* Cambridge, MA Harvard University Press 1991.

Mann, John *Murder, Magic and Medicine* Oxford Oxford University Press 1994.

Manniche, Lise *An Ancient Egyptian Herbal* London British Museum Publications 1989.

Mendlesohn, Everett *Heat and Life* Cambridge, MA Harvard University Press 1964.

Meulenbeld, G.J. "The Many Faces of Ayurveda" *Journal of the European Ayurvedic Society*, vol. 4 1995 pp. 1-10.

Meulenbeld, G.J., Wujastyk, D. (editors) *Studies On Indian Medical History* Groningen Egbert Forsten 1987.

Mills, Simon *Out of the Earth* London Viking-Penguin 1991

Newman Turner, Roger *Naturopathic Medicine* Wellinborough Thorsons 1990.

Neuburger, Max *The Doctrine of the Healing Power of Nature Throughout the Course of Time* trasnslated by L.J. Boyd New York (privately printed) 1932.

Nutton, V. "Humoralism" in Bynum, W.F. and Porter, R. (eds.) *Companion Encyclopedia of the History of Medicine* London Routledge 1993 pp. 281-291.

Nutton, V. *From Democedes to Harvey: Studies in the history of medicine from the Greeks to the renaissance* London Variorum 1988.

Onians, Richard Broxton *The Origins of European Thought about the Body, the Mind, the Soul, the World, Time and Fate* Cambridge Cambridge University Press 1951.

Phillips, E.D. *Greek Medicine* London Thames and Hudson 1973.

Pietroni, Patrick *The Greening of Medicine* London Victor Gollancz 1990.

Porter, Roy *The Greatest Benefit to Mankind* London Harper Colins 1997.

Riddle, J.M. *Dioscorides on Pharmacy and Medicine* Austin, TX University of Texas Press 1985.

Sallares, R. *The Ecology of the Ancient Greek World* London Duckworth 1991.

Sambursky, S. *The Physical World of the Greeks* Jerusalem Hebrew University Press, London Routledge and Kegan Paul 1963.

Sedlar, Jean W. *India and the Greek World* Totowa NJ Rowona and Littlefields 1980.

Seyle, Hans, M.D. *The Stress of Life* London McGraw-Hill 1978.

Sharan, Farida *Herbs of Grace* Boulder, CO Wisdome Press 1989.

Siegel, R. *Galen's System of Physiology and Medicine* Basel and New York Karger 1968.

Sigerist, Henry E. *A History of Medicine, Vol II. Early Greek Hindu and Persian Medicine* Oxford, Oxford University Press 1987.

Solmsen, F. "The Vital Heat, The inborn *pneuma* and the *Aether" Journal of Hellenic Studies* 77 1957 pp. 119-123.

Smith, W.D. *The Hippocratic Tradition* Ithaca NY Cornell University Press 1979.

Smith, W.D. *Hippocrates: Pseudographic Writings* Leiden E.J. Brill 1990.

Smutts, J. *Holism and Evolution* London Macmillan 1926.

Svoboda, Robert *Ayurveda, Life, Health and Longevity* London Penguin Books/Arkana 1992.

Taylor, H.O. *Greek Biology and Medicine* New York Cooper Square Inc. 1963.

Tempin O., Tempin C.L. (eds.) *Ancient Medicine: Selected papers of Ludwig Edelstein* Baltimore and London Johns Hopkins University Press 1967.

Thivel, A. *Cnide et Cos?* essai surles doctrines medicals dans hippocratique Peris Les belles lettres 1981.

Tierra, Michael *The Way of Herbs* Santa Cruz, CA Orenda-Unity Press 1980.

Temkin, O. *Hippocrates in a World of Pagans and Christians* Baltimore and London Johns Hopkins University Press 1995.

Tobyn, Graeme *Culpeper's Medicine, A Practice of Western Holistic Medicine* Shaftesbury Dorset Element Books 1997.

van der Kroon, Coen *Beneath the Surface of the Body: Life Force and Female-Male Polarity, A structural approach to Hippocratic gynecology with concepts from eastern medicine* unpublished thesis submitted to the State University of Groningen 1989.

van der Eijk, P. J., Horstmashoff, H.F., Schrijvers, P.H., (eds.) *Ancient Medicine in its Socio-Cultural Context* vols. I, II. Amsterdam and Atlanta Rodopi 1995.

Vlastos, G. "Theology and Philosophy in Early Greek Thought" *Philosophical Quarterly* II 97-123 published in *Studies in Pre-Socratic Philosophy* 2 vols. London 1970 and 1975

Vogel, H.C. *Nature Doctor* Edinburgh Mainstream Publishing Co. 1982.

von Staden, Heinrich *Herophilus, The Art of Medicine in Early Alexandria* Cambridge Cambridge University Press 1989.

Voswinckel, P. "Black bile in the doctrine of the four humours. New empirical aspects" in Fierens E., Tricot J-P., Appelboom T., Thierry M. (eds.) *Proceedings of the XXXIInd International Congress on the History of Medicine* Antwerp 3-7 September 1990 Bruxeles [Belgium] Societas Belgica Historiac Medicine 1991.

West, M.L. *The Orphic Poems* Oxford The Clarendon Press 1983.

West, M.L. *Early Greek Philosophy and the Orient* Oxford The Clarendon Press 1971.

Wheeler, R.E.M. *Five Thousand Years of Pakistan* London Royal India and Pakistan Society 1950.

Wheeler, Sir Mortimer *Civilisations of the Indus Valley and Beyond* London Thames and Hudson 1966.

Wilkins, John, Harvey, David and Dodson, Mike (eds.) *Food in Antiquity: Studies in Ancient Society and Culture* Exeter Exeter University Press 1995.

Woodcock, George *The Marvellous Century: Archaic Man and the Awakening of Reason* Markham, Ontario Fitzhenry and Whiteside 1989.

*World Health Organisation Programmes* http://www.who.org/programmes/dap/trmO.html. 1997.

Wujastyk, Dominik *The Roots of Ayurveda, Selections from Sanskrit Medical Writings* New Delhi Penguin, India 1998; London Penguin New edn. 2003.

Zysk, Kenneth G. *Asceticism and Healing in Ancient India* Oxford Oxford University Press 1991.

# INDEX

digestive residues and 113
emotions and 121
excess and 111
explanations of 20
external factors 164-5
humoral theory 4
internal factors 165
pathological digestion and 129-31
*pneuma* and 114-15
stages of 163-5
stress and 62, 120
supernatural and 3, 18
taste and 104-5
theory of 14
vital force and 53-4, 76
*Diseases I* 148, 181, 187
on humours 176-7, 190-1, 192-3
*Diseases II* 192
*Diseases III* 124
*Diseases IV* 191, 201
on humours 156, 175, 176, 183, 188, 197, 204
*Diseases of Women* 88
divine force 47-52
*doṣas* xiv, 164
formed by elements 158-63
imbalance in 163, 167
location of 160-1
mental 161, 162
movement of 161, 162-63, 169
*prakṛti* and 165, 167
and seasons 163, 200
similarities with humours 206-11
see also *kapha; pitta; vāta*
dreams 45, 88, 119-20
dropsy 191, 192
drugs 66, 67, 72-3, 106, 167
*dunameis* 4, 9, 15, 87

## E

East-West College of Herbalism (Sussex, England) 140
Edelstein, Ludwig 7, 22
elimination 97
embryology 84, 128, 201, 210
emetic therapy 122, 137, 138
emetics 66, 88, 99, 100, 120, 130
emotions 55, 58-9, 121
Empedocles of Acragas 13, 101
on blood 14-15, 102
and elements 8, 49, 85, 192, 197, 198, 205-6
enemas 99-100
*Epidemics* 14, 107, 123, 182
on humours 178, 181, 183, 188, 189, 193, 195
on mind-body relationship 50, 55, 56, 120, 196
on nature 51-2
on treatments 67-8, 84, 88, 123
epilepsy 57, 196
causes of 63, 117, 119, 166, 180, 190, 195, 203, 207
Eryximachus 23, 43, 206
essential oil therapy 183, 214
Euryphon 113-14
excess 179-80
in Āyurveda 137-9, 162, 163
in Hippocratic *Corpus* 111-12, 136-7
exercise 91, 167, 176
and food 86-7, 88, 98-9
as treatment 66, 120, 136-7
existence, explanation of 35

## F

Fahraeus, Robin 194
fasting 93, 114, 117, 121-2, 125, 131, 139
Featherstone, Cornelia xxiii-xxiv
fevers 20, 54, 73, 164, 187
and bile 187
treatments for 68-9, 114, 121-6, 131-4
Filliozat, Jean xvi, 25, 33, 144, 170-1
flatulence 105, 113
*Fleshes* 103, 155, 184, 197
folk traditions 149

similarities with *doṣas* 206-11 –
and therapeutic methods 181-3
and tissue formation 85-6
*see* also bile; blood; *doṣas;* melancholy; phlegm; water
*Humours* 57, 61-2, 84, 180, 199
disease, causes of 63, 119, 120, 182
hydromel 96

I

immunology 216
incantations 27, 73
India xiv, 24
society 36-41
individuals, and disease 62, 74
infections 20
inflammations 20
innate heat 91-2, 100-1, 153
*Internal affections* 84, 124, 186, 191, 192, 199
International Workshop on the Study of Indian Medicine xvi
Isvarakrisna 34

J

Jainism 31, 39
*jala* 157, 160
jaundice 28-9
*jñānendriyāṇi* 35
Jolly, Julius xvi, 24, 159
Joly, Robert 145-6
Jones, W.H.S. 2, 19, 88, 89-90, 145, 195
on malaria 193-4
on treatments 121, 123
Jouanna, Jacques 146
*Journal of the European Ayurvedic Society* xvi

K

*kapha* 35, 133, 137-8, 163, 168, 169, 200
characteristics of 160, 162, 164
site of 137, 161
*karmendriyāṇi* 35
*katastasis* 180, 183
*kosmos* 8-9, 13, 51
*krasis* 18, 84-5, 87, 90, 92, 93
Kuhn, Thomas 3, 4

L

Lain Entralgo, Pedro 147, 150-1
laughter therapy 60, 179
*Law* 52
*Law of Manu* 36, 37
Leucippus 49
lifestyle 57, 63
Littré, M.P.E. xvi
liver 102, 174
Lloyd, G.E.R. 7, 8, 19, 146
*logismos* 87-8
Longrigg, James 3, 8, 19, 101
Lonie, Iain 148-9, 156, 192
Luce, J.V. 11

M

madness 198, 204: *see also* melancholia
magico-religious approach to health 27, 28, 41-2
*mahābhūtas* 35
*mahat* 35
Mahavira 28, 33, 39
malaria 193-4
man, nature of 13, 147-50, 153-4, 155
*manas* 35
manipulation xviii
mantra techniques 214
marrow 102, 103, 174, 184
massage therapies xvii n. 11, xviii, 66, 67, 214
medical reasoning 150-2, 181
medicine:
and philosophy 17-20
and spiritual knowledge 74-6
tastes and 105-6